Health Policy and Federalism

A Comparative Perspective on Multi-Level Governance

D0167519

Social Union Series

Federalism, Democracy and Labour Market Policy in Canada,
Tom McIntosh, editor

Federalism, Democracy and Health Policy in Canada, Duane Adams, editor

*Disability and Federalism: Comparing Different Approaches to Full
Participation,* David Cameron and Fraser Valentine, editors

*Health Policy and Federalism: A Comparative Perspective on Multi-Level
Governance,* Keith G. Banting and Stan Corbett, editors

Health Policy and Federalism

A Comparative Perspective on Multi-Level Governance

EDITED BY KEITH G. BANTING
AND STAN CORBETT

Published for the Institute of Intergovernmental Relations
School of Policy Studies, Queen's University
by McGill-Queen's University Press
Montreal & Kingston • London • Ithaca

National Library of Canada Cataloguing in Publication Data

Main entry under title:

Health policy and federalism : a comparative perspective on multi-level governance

(Social union series)
Includes bibliographical references.
ISBN 1-55339-000-8 (bound).—ISBN 0-88911-589-0 (pbk.)

1. Medical policy. 2. Federal government. I. Banting, Keith G., 1947- II. Corbett, S. M. (Stanley M.), 1945- III. Queen's University (Kingston, Ont.). Institute of Intergovernmental Relations. IV. Series.

RA393.H42 2001   362.1   C2001-903952-2

The Institute of Intergovernmental Relations

The Institute is the only organization in Canada whose mandate is solely to promote research and communication on the challenges facing the federal system.

Current research interests include fiscal federalism, the social union, the reform of federal political institutions and the machinery of federal-provincial relations, Canadian federalism and the global economy, and comparative federalism.

The Institute pursues these objectives through research conducted by its own staff and other scholars, through its publication program, and through seminars and conferences.

The Institute links academics and practitioners of federalism in federal and provincial governments and the private sector.

The Institute of Intergovernmental Relations receives ongoing financial support from the J.A. Corry Memorial Endowment Fund, the Royal Bank of Canada Endowment Fund, Power Corporation, the Government of Canada, and the Government of Ontario. We are grateful for this support which enables the Institute to sustain its extensive program of research, publication, and related activities.

L'Institut des relations intergouvernementales

L'Institut est le seul organisme canadien à se consacrer exclusivement à la recherche et aux échanges sur les questions du fédéralisme.

Les priorités de recherche de l'Institut portent présentement sur le fédéralisme fiscal, l'union sociale, la modification éventuelle des institutions politiques fédérales, les nouveaux mécanismes de relations fédérales-provinciales, le fédéralisme canadien au regard de l'économie mondiale et le fédéralisme comparatif.

L'Institut réalise ses objectifs par le biais de recherches effectuées par son personnel et par des universitaires de l'Université Queen's et d'ailleurs, de même que par des conférences et des colloques.

L'Institut sert de lien entre les universitaires, les fonctionnaires fédéraux et provinciaux et le secteur privé.

L'institut des relations intergouvernementales reçoit l'appui financier du J.A. Corry Memorial Endowment Fund, de la Fondation de la Banque Royale du Canada, de Power Corporation, du gouvernement du Canada et du gouvernement de l'Ontario. Nous les remercions de cet appui qui permet à l'Institut de poursuivre son vaste programme de recherche et de publication ainsi que ses activités connexes.

CONTENTS

INTRODUCTION TO SERIES

This is one of six volumes being published by the Institute of Intergovernmental Relations related to the Canadian Social Union. Three of the volumes compare the way in which different federations handle various aspects of social policy. These volumes, including this one edited by Keith G. Banting and Stan Corbett, will be of interest to those who study comparative federalism and comparative health and social policy. The other three volumes are based on a series of case studies of how Canadian governments manage intergovernmental relations in particular areas of health and social programming.

The work for this series began in 1997, well before the 1999 signing of the Social Union Framework Agreement. Even at that time, as a result of the substantial cuts in federal fiscal transfers to the provinces, it seemed that a new set of relationships was going to be required between federal and provincial governments in order to improve both the quality of social policy in Canada and the health of the federation.

In conceiving of the volumes for this series, two considerations were paramount. The first was that there was relatively little empirical literature on the way in which federal and provincial governments relate to one another, and to citizens and interest groups, in designing and delivering social programs. Yet it is at the level of programs and citizens, as much as at the level of political symbolism and high politics, that the social union is in practice defined. To help fill this knowledge gap, we thought it appropriate to design a series of case studies on the governance of Canadian social programs. And to ensure that the results of the case studies could be compared to one another, the Institute developed a research methodology that authors were asked to take into account as they conducted their research. This methodology built on earlier work by Margaret Biggs in analyzing these governance relationships from the perspective of their impact on policy, federalism, and democracy.

The second consideration was that Canadians were insufficiently aware of how other federations handle these same kinds of social program relationships. As a result, we thought it important to recruit authors from different federations who could explain the governance of social policy in their countries. This volume thus compares the way in which five different federations deal with health policy.

While the research for these volumes was under way, a series of roundtables and workshops (nine in total) was held. Those invited included officials from provincial and federal governments, representatives from stakeholder groups and individuals from the research community as well the case study authors. The purpose of these roundtables and workshops was to review and comment on the Canadian and comparative case studies. I thank the numerous participants in these events for helping the authors and editors with their work.

This series received financial assistance from the federal government (Health Canada and Human Resources Development Canada) and the governments of New Brunswick, Ontario, Saskatchewan and Alberta. An advisory committee that included officials from these same jurisdictions as well as from academe also assisted in the development of the project. In fact, it was this committee that helped in the selection of the three sectors that are the subject of this series: health, disability, and labour market.

The 1999 Social Union Framework Agreement is open for review early in 2002. The agreement states that this review process will "ensure significant opportunities for input and feedback from Canadians..." It is hoped that this series will constitute a significant input to that process.

Harvey Lazar
General Editor
Social Union Series

ACKNOWLEDGEMENTS

This book has been shaped by the ideas, energy and enthusiasm of many people. Its origins lie in the ambitious project launched by the Institute of Intergovernmental Relations to study the ways in which federal states manage the complexities of multi-level governance in the field of social policy. We would like to thank Harvey Lazar and his colleagues in the Institute for the opportunity to contribute to the project, for their support along the way, and for their patience with the seemingly endless editorial process.

We would also like to thank the authors for their thoughtful analyses of the complex interactions between federal institutions and health policy in their own countries. Initial drafts of the country chapters were presented at a workshop held at Queen's University. The authors, editors and a number of officials from the health sector discussed the papers and debated the subtle relations between political institutions and policy outcomes in federal states. The discussions and suggestions that flowed from those conversations enhanced the quality of the book in important ways.

Finally, we would like to thank the Publications Unit at the School of Policy Studies. They coped masterfully with the challenges posed by authors spread out over three continents, and by editors who brought an unforgiveable inattentiveness to many of the imperatives of an efficient publication process.

Keith G. Banting and Stan Corbett
December 2001

CONTRIBUTORS

KEITH G. BANTING, School of Policy Studies, Queen's University, Kingston

DAVID C. COLBY, The Robert Wood Johnson Foundation, Princeton

STAN CORBETT, Faculty of Law and Department of Philosophy, Queen's University, Kingston

JOHAN DE COCK, The National Sickness and Invalidity Insurance Institute (NSIII), Brussels

LINDA HANCOCK, Public Policy and Governance Program, Deakin University, Melbourne

ANTONIA MAIONI, McGill Institute for the Study of Canada/Institut d'études canadiennes de McGill, McGill University, Montreal

DIETMAR WASSENER, Gesellschaft für Datenverarbeitung GmbH (Pharmafakt), Munich/Bavaria

1

HEALTH POLICY AND FEDERALISM: AN INTRODUCTION

Keith G. Banting and Stan Corbett

Governments everywhere are wrestling with health policy.[1] They must balance the needs and expectations of citizens, the demands of health-care professionals and the pressures on public budgets; and everywhere the trade-offs are becoming more difficult. In federal countries, these challenges are met through political institutions that require the participation and cooperation of at least two levels of government in the design and redesign of health policy, adding another layer of complexity to the management of health policies. This study examines the ways in which different federal systems manage the tensions inherent in multi-level governance, and the implications of federalism for the nature of health programs.

The analysis is based on a comparative study of the experience of five federations: Australia, Belgium, Canada, Germany, and the United States, which are examined in detail in the chapters that follow. However, the implications of the study extend beyond these five countries. Indeed, the historic distinction between federal and unitary states is blurring at the edges as traditionally unitary systems such as Britain and Italy experiment with new forms of regional government, and a wide range of countries devolve important policy responsibilities to a diverse range of regional assemblies and administrations. Although important differences remain between federations and devolved systems of governance, many of the political dynamics and policy issues generated by these differing forms of multi-level governance are remarkably similar, and a closer study of health care in federal states therefore has broader lessons.[2]

A comparative approach establishes a much stronger basis for assessing the policy consequences of distinctive political institutions. Too often, analysts and commentators casually assume that the inability of their own political leaders to solve pressing policy problems must reflect flaws in the political institutions and processes of their country. Most often, however, other countries are wrestling with remarkably similar problems, usually with equally mixed results. A comparative perspective can help identify what is truly distinctive about a country, and provide a much stronger starting point for attempting to assess the policy consequences of any particular configuration of political institutions. This study employs a variety of methodologies to highlight these relationships. It draws on insights from the wider literature on the influence of political structures; it presents quantitative comparisons of federal and nonfederal states; and it utilizes a "most similar systems" approach to comparative analysis. This last technique involves the comparison of countries that share many similarities — federal institutions, relatively affluent economies, and common pressures on their health-care systems — in order to pinpoint the influence of variation in the nature of their federal institutions. In all of the federations surveyed here, both levels of government are involved in shaping health policy. There are, however, important differences in the form of their federal arrangements and in the design of their health-care systems. It is the interactions between these distinctive political institutions and health care that lie at the heart of this study.

This introductory chapter provides an overview of the issues and seeks to draw out the patterns that emerge from the country chapters for several critical policy issues. The first section briefly summarizes the common health-care agenda confronted by governments across the Organisation for Economic Co-operation and Development (OECD). The second section sets the context for the analysis by examining the wider literature on the implications of federalism and by asking whether federal and non-federal countries differ systematically in their broad approach to health policy. The third section shifts the focus more directly onto the five federations explored here, describing their federal institutions and the ways in which decisions about health policy are made. The fourth section then examines the implications of their federal structures for two basic policy challenges: citizens' access to health services and the effectiveness of strategies deployed to contain the growth of health-care expenditures. A final section then pulls the threads of the discussion together.

As we shall see, these threads are quite strong. While federalism is clearly compatible with a wide range of health-care systems, the presence of federal institutions does seem to influence the balance between the public and private sectors in the provision of health care. In addition, differences in intergovernmental arrangements within federations have potent implications for such issues as the equality of health services enjoyed by citizens across the country as a whole, and the capacity of governments to manage health-care systems efficiently.

A COMMON AGENDA

Health policy is a salient issue in virtually every OECD country, and the governments of these countries — federal and non-federal alike — confront a remarkably similar health agenda. In part, this common agenda reflects similar policy goals. In its 1999 *World Health Report*, the World Health Organization set out a list of six core health goals: improving the health status of the population; reducing health inequalities; enhancing responsiveness to legitimate expectations; increasing efficiency of the health-care delivery systems; protecting individuals, families, and communities from significant financial loss as a result of health problems; and enhancing fairness in the financing and delivery of health care.[3] Different countries, including the five examined here, have developed very different approaches to health care, with different public/ private mixes, different relationships among service providers, and different delivery systems. Nevertheless, few, if any, of those involved in health policy in these countries would find much to disagree with in this core list of goals.

The shared agenda in health care also reflects the fact that OECD countries face a common set of pressures: aging populations, rapid technological change, rising health expenditures, changing understandings of the determinants of health, and a more nuanced appreciation of the relationship between health care and health outcomes. Moreover, in most countries, governments must respond to these pressures in the context of fiscal constraint. Although the public sector has moved into surplus in some countries, international economic competitiveness and domestic political resistance to high levels of taxation mean that few governments can manage the challenges in the health sector by simply opening their wallets wider.

Common goals, common pressures and common constraints have generated a shared agenda. Governments throughout the OECD debate a remarkably similar set of issues: the provision of quality health care; cost containment through a mix of price controls, volume controls and/or global budgeting; new incentive structures for health professionals through changes in payment systems; shifts in the public/private mix in health services; responses to rapidly escalating pharmaceutical costs; the need for innovation and flexibility in delivery systems; provision for long-term care and support for the frail elderly; and greater accountability to, and empowerment of, the public. These are the familiar points of discussion among health policy specialists across western, democratic countries. The issue in this study is whether federal institutions matter to the ways in which our five countries respond.

DOES FEDERALISM MAKE A DIFFERENCE?

There is a substantial body of literature that explores the extent to which political institutions influence the types of policies that emerge at the end of the day. The broad conclusion that flows from this new "institutionalist" approach is that political institutions alone are never determinative. They interact with other factors shaping policy choices, and it is therefore difficult to identify simple relationships of the sort "federal institutions lead to X." Nevertheless, the structures of government are seldom completely neutral. They make some outcomes easier than others, and therefore influence the capacity of political agents to act, their perceptions of realistic policy alternatives, their strategic options, and their preferences.[4] Studies have suggested that, in combination with other factors, the configuration of political institutions can matter to such things as the size of the public sector, the redistributive role of government, the level of coherence across programs, the interregional distribution of benefits across the country, the level of innovation and flexibility in the policy system, the capacity of governments to resist powerful interests, and so on.

Given the contingent nature of the impact of political institutions, one should not expect to find powerful patterns between such broad categories as federal versus non-federal countries. For example, in their basic approach to the welfare state, the five countries examined here fall into three or more of the regime clusters proposed by Esping-Andersen and extended by others.[5] Nor does a more consistent pattern emerge when attention is narrowed to the health-care system. As we shall see in greater detail below, our five countries have developed very different regimes of health care. Belgium and Germany have comprehensive health-care systems in which policy is defined through corporatist systems of decision-making and services are managed and delivered locally through networks of social funds. Australia and Canada have developed comprehensive public health insurance programs that are managed by public agencies. And the United States has developed a unique mixed system in which public programs cover the elderly, the disabled and many low-income families, while the rest of the population relies on private coverage and a significant minority lack coverage. The basic structure of health care is clearly rooted in other factors, such as the political culture and the dominant political coalitions in each country, with the particular configuration of political institutions playing a decidedly secondary role.[6]

Federal institutions do seem to have implications, however, for the size of the public role in the health sector. This pattern is consistent with a substantial body of research that concludes that federalism and decentralization tended to constrain the expansion of the welfare state during the twentieth century. A large number of studies have concluded that federalism and decentralization create several types of barriers that constrain an expansive and redistributive welfare state: by increasing the number of sites of political representation, federalism multiplies the number of veto points at which action can be delayed, diluted, or defeated; by creating separate regional jurisdictions, federalism generates interregional economic competition as state/provincial governments compete for private capital, which can exit for other regions with more hospitable fiscal regimes. These arguments have been advanced in numerous studies of individual federations.[7] Although the completeness of the evidence deployed in such studies has been criticized,[8] the argument gains strong additional support from a substantial body of quantitative, cross-national studies of the determinants of social spending. These studies have identified a variety of factors that help explain differences in the expansiveness of the welfare state across OECD nations, including the openness of the economy, the strength of organized labour, and the ideological orientation of dominant political parties. This literature has increasingly focused on the structure of political institutions, and findings repeatedly indicate that, other things being equal, the dispersion of policy-making authority through federalism, decentralization, and other forms of institutional fragmentation is negatively associated with social expenditures as a proportion of gross domestic product (GDP).[9] Moreover, a recent contribution to this literature finds that decentralization has more powerful (negative) effects on social welfare effort even than other institutional variables, such as the level of corporatism in decision-making, the nature of the electoral system or the presence of a presidential system of government.[10] In addition, new research that approaches the issue from the other side of the ledger by examining the private share of overall social expenditures in OECD nations comes to similar conclusions.[11]

What about the health-care sector in particular? As Table 1 indicates, total health expenditure, including both public and private spending, actually tends to be higher in federal than non-federal states. However, when attention focuses on the balance between the public and private sector in health care, the pattern that emerges is consistent with the conclusions of the cross-national literature. Table 1, which also examines the balance between public and private expenditures on health in 1998, indicates that public spending represented a smaller percentage of total health expenditures in federal states than in non-federal ones (an average of 70.3 percent versus 79.1 percent). This result is influenced to some extent by the United States, where public spending represents an especially small proportion of total health expenditures, but it does not disappear when the United States is excluded from the calculations: public spending averages 74.6 percent of total health expenditures in all OECD federal states minus the United States, versus the 79.1 percent in non-federal OECD states.

TABLE 1
Health Expenditures in Federal and Non-Federal States, 1998

	Total *as % GDP*	*Public* *as % of Total*	*Private* *as % of Total*
Australia	8.5	69.3	30.7
Belgium	8.8	89.7	10.3
Canada	9.5	69.6	30.4
Germany	10.6	74.6	25.4
United States	13.6	44.7	55.3
Average	10.2	69.6	30.4
OECD			
OECD Average	8.5	76.2	23.8
Non-federal	7.8	79.1	20.9
Federal	9.9	70.3	29.7
Federal–US	9.3	74.6	25.4

Note: In these calculations, OECD Federal states include Australia, Austria, Belgium, Canada, Germany, Switzerland, and the United States. OECD Non-Federal states include Denmark, Finland, France, Iceland, Ireland, Italy, Japan, Luxembourg, Netherlands, New Zealand, Norway, Spain, Sweden, and the United Kingdom.

Source: Organisation for Economic Co-operation and Development, *OECD Health Data 2000: A Comparative Analysis of 29 Countries* (Paris: OECD).

Figure 1 puts this difference in a longer term perspective by tracking the data from 1960 to 1998 (for more detail, see also Table A1). The difference between federal and non-federal states is a long-standing one, but one that has been decreasing over time. The data on the rates of change in Table A1 provide some clues to this partial convergence: the public share of total health spending grew more rapidly in federal states during the 1960s, narrowing to some extent the gap generated by the earlier expansion of the public role in non-federal states; and then federal states did not constrain the public share during the 1980s and 1990s as sharply as did non-federal states. One interpretation of this pattern is that the complexity of decision-making in federal states means that they tend to react more slowly to new conditions than do non-federal states. If so, one might expect the pattern of convergence to slow, as federal states develop stronger instruments of cost containment over time.

These differences in spending patterns are intriguing, and we return to some of the issues they pose below in our discussion of the challenges that

FIGURE 1
Public Expenditure as Percent of Total Health Expenditures, Federal and Non-Federal States, 1960–1998

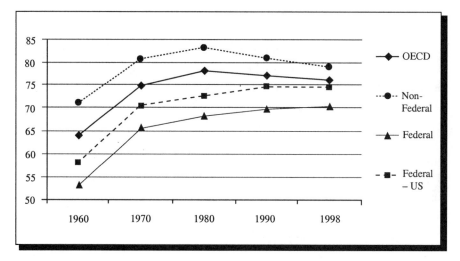

Notes: For Federal and Non-Federal, see notes to Table 1. German data in 1990s include east Germany.

Source: OECD, *OECD Health Data 2000.*

TABLE 2
Population Health Status in Federal and Non-Federal States

	Life Expectancy	*Infant Mortality*	*Ranking of Population Health*	*Ranking of Health System Performance*
Australia	78.3	5	39	32
Belgium	77.3	6	28	21
Canada	79.1	6	35	30
Germany	77.3	5	41	25
United States	76.8	7	72	37
Average	77.8	6		
OECD				
OECD	77.8	5		
Federal	77.8	5.5		
Non-Federal	77.8	5		

Notes: For Federal and Non-Federal see the Notes to Table 1. Columns 1 and 2 are for 1998; columns 3 and 4 are for 1997, and represent rankings out of 191 countries by the World Health Organization.

Sources: Columns 1 and 2: *United Nations Human Development Report 2000*; columns 3 and 4 are from the *World Health Report 2000*.

federal states face in coping with cost pressures in the health sector. However, such spending variations represent only incremental variations on the basic patterns of health care in OECD countries, and the simple contrast between federal and non-federal regimes only takes one so far. Certainly, as Table 2 confirms, there is no reason to believe that institutional differences make an appreciable difference to the overall health of populations within states at broadly comparable stages of economic development. A fuller and more nuanced understanding of the interactions between federalism and health care requires an examination of the experience of specific federal countries.

FEDERALISM AND HEALTH POLICY: FIVE CASES

A closer look at federal institutions highlights that there is no single model of federalism. Indeed, in the words of one analyst, "perhaps the most intellectually endearing quality of federalism" is that there is "an eclectic array of federal political models ... from which other states may draw lessons and experience as they choose."[12] The five federations examined in this study differ considerably in the role of federal and state or provincial governments in health care, the ways in which decisions about health policy are made, and the mechanisms for coordinating relations between different orders of government. It is hardly surprising, therefore, that federalism does not influence health policy similarly in all countries.

There is a myriad of ways in which one can compare federal institutions.[13] A common approach is to assess the level of centralization between the central and state/provincial governments by measuring the proportion of public expenditures or revenues flowing through each level of government. This fiscal approach to federalism has important advantages beyond mere quantitative precision. Money is power, and command over resources does influence the political balance between levels of government in federations. However, finances represent an incomplete measure of the policy role of different levels of governments. Given the focus in this study, a better measure is the role of different levels of government in defining the basic framework of health policy. Are the core features of a health-care regime set centrally or regionally? This question cannot be answered in precise, quantifiable terms, but it is the heart of the matter. If the basic elements of the health-care system are set centrally, then whether actual expenditures are made locally is a secondary question. In this chapter, therefore, two questions are critical. First, how specific is the country-wide framework for health-care policy? Does it resolve most of the important decisions, or does it leave substantial scope for regional variation? Second, how is the central framework determined? Is it set unilaterally by the central government or do state/provincial governments have an important role in its determination as well? In answering these questions, we draw heavily on the country chapters that make up the heart of this volume, and readers are referred to those chapters for fuller details.

Because our analysis draws on two distinct criteria — the comprehensiveness of the central framework and the process of its determination — no simple rank order of centralization is possible. In presenting our five cases, we start with the countries with the most comprehensive and detailed central frameworks. In the case of countries with comparable common frameworks, we first examine countries in which the central government has the greatest independence in setting that framework.

Belgium

Although Belgium was established in 1830 as a unitary state, four major waves of constitutional reform in 1970, 1980, 1988, and 1993 created a decentralized federal state, with substantial powers exercised by the new Community and Regional governments. Moreover, a new wave of constitutional reform was launched in 2001. Despite this dramatic restructuring of state structures, however, primary responsibility for social security and health care remains lodged in the central government. The federal government retains exclusive responsibility for health insurance, and sets the framework within which local sickness funds function. In addition, Brussels establishes framework legislation for health-care institutions such as hospitals, setting regulations for planning, accreditation, staffing, equipment, advanced technology and the designation of academic hospitals. According to the calculations in the chapter by Johan de Cock, approximately 97 percent of total health-care expenditures remain in areas of federal jurisdiction. The Communities do have a role in the construction and internal organization of hospitals, and for the organization and management of home care and nursing homes.[14] However, they are constrained by federal norms or financing policies in many of these areas and must communicate their decisions — including those pertaining to individual cases — to the central authorities who are responsible for ensuring that central norms are respected. Only in public health and medical education is Community authority dominant.

Although power remains highly centralized in health care, policy-making within the federal government is subject to the elaborate consultative mechanisms of corporatist governance that characterize the Belgian political system. Three dimensions of *concertation* are relevant. Major policy decisions require the consent of federal representatives from both the French- and Flemish-speaking groups. In addition, although the Regional and Community governments have no formal role in the federal legislature, an elaborate set of rules and regulations in the health sector mandate notification and consultation between levels of government. Finally, consultative mechanisms incorporate the social partners and the medical professions into the policy process. As a result, changes in health programs require high levels of consensus among both linguistic blocs and social groups.

Despite this consultative tradition, the highly centralized nature of health policy in Belgium has come under powerful pressure as a result of the growth of Flemish nationalism. Flemish nationalists have demanded significant decentralization of key elements of social security, including health insurance, in order to gain more control over their social future and to reform the inter-communal transfers inherent in the currently centralized system, demands that have been articulated by the new Flemish parliament. However, determined resistance from the Wallonian community to decentralization of social security has blocked such changes and, for the moment at least, Belgian health care represents a centralized corner of a decentralized, binational state.

Germany

As in the case of Belgium, federalism plays a secondary role in health policy in Germany. As the chapter by Dietmar Wassener makes clear, the framework for health programs is set, with few exceptions, through federal legislation that applies evenly across the country. The basic features of this framework are defined through highly corporatist processes that incorporate not only representatives of the social partners — such as employers and employees, health professionals and social funds — but also both levels of government. The Länder governments are directly involved in the federal legislative process through the Bundersrat, the upper level of the federal parliament, and establishing the parameters of health policy therefore requires a high level of intergovernmental consensus.

The legislative framework established in this way defines the core features of the statutory system of health insurance, which covers over 90 percent of the population. The framework sets: minimum standards for health services; the principles governing contribution rates, including maximum rates; and maximum budgets for the hospital sector, ambulatory care, and pharmaceuticals. Within this common framework, the specific design and delivery of health services are highly decentralized, being the responsibility of close to 600 independent social funds. These funds are managed by representatives of employers and employees, and the services they provide are financed by contributions from employers and employees rather than tax revenues from the state. Within the national parameters, the funds decide on the precise health services they will cover, set their contribution rates, and negotiate contracts with associations representing doctors and hospitals. As a result, the direct delivery responsibilities of governments are limited. The Länder governments do have responsibility for public health promotion and for financing the capital costs of hospitals. This last provision produces a dual source of financing for hospitals, with the Länder providing for capital costs and the social funds providing the bulk of operating costs, a division that occasionally produces conflict between the two. Nevertheless, in the parlance of new public management, the primary function of government in health care is steering, not rowing.

In such a system, it is hard to define precisely where leadership ultimately comes from. Decisions to reform the statutory health insurance system are taken at the national level, and are normally led by the federal government, usually in concert with state governments controlled by the same party. However, their proposals tend to be modified during negotiations with representatives of the funds and provider associations, and during passage through the upper house. Indeed, the process requires such a high level of intergovernmental and social consensus that critics, including Wassener, complain of an institutionalized rigidity and inflexibility that constrains policy-making in a rapidly changing world.[15]

Australia

Federalism is more central to the politics of health care in Australia, but once again the federal government plays the leading role in setting the basic parameters of health policy, as Linda Hancock's chapter demonstrates. A 1946 constitutional amendment extended the Commonwealth's powers to include laws on pharmaceutical, sickness and hospital benefits, and medical and dental services. As a result, Medicare, the national health program established in 1984, is delivered in two parts, one purely federal and the other federal/state in design. The Commonwealth government provides directly for access to doctors, pharmaceuticals, and nursing homes under the Medical Benefits and Pharmaceutical Benefits Schemes, which are administered by the Commonwealth's Health Insurance Commission and operate on similar terms across the entire country.

In contrast, access to public hospital care is established through bilateral Commonwealth/state agreements, which are renegotiated every five years. However, the Commonwealth government exerts considerable influence here as well, and hospital care preserves the characteristics of a common "national" service. The primary instruments of federal influence are Special Purpose Payments (SPPs), grants to states that are subject to conditions aimed at ensuring compliance with national goals. The main SPP in the hospital sector, known as the Health Care Grant, is ringed with highly detailed requirements; for example, all public hospitals in the states are expected to comply with performance targets set by the Commonwealth Department for Health and Family Services, which constantly audits to ensure that the targets are met. During the 1980s, the reliance on the conditional SPPs did shift as a result of changes in the government in power in Canberra, with Labor governments favouring conditional grants and Liberal/National coalitions tipping the balance more toward unconditional block grants. Since then, however, the role of SPPs has been reinstated as a continuing source of central influence on hospital care, and even conservative administrations have shown little inclination to relax conditions attached to federal social program funding. In addition, as the chapter on Australia by Linda Hancock indicates, the Commonwealth government influences health services through initiatives that cover government services as a whole, such as its National Competition Policy.

Although the parameters of health policy therefore tend to be set centrally, state governments have opportunities to influence the federal framework through the complex set of intergovernmental bodies that characterize Australian federalism. The Commonwealth Grants Commission, which is jointly appointed by the two levels of government, plays a critical role in managing intergovernmental conflicts over financial issues. In addition, the Premiers' Conferences, ministerial conferences, the Loans Council and, in recent years, the Council of Australian Governments (COAG) represent sites of intergovernmental negotiation in which important initiatives are developed jointly and intergovernmental conflicts managed. The Commonwealth government tends to provide the leadership within these bodies, but the network of institutions does provide for regular debate and coordination between levels of government. Although these mechanisms of intergovernmental coordination are not as powerful as in the German case, they do ensure that many social programs are guided by national, as well as more narrowly federal objectives.

United States

The United States resembles Australia in relying on separate federal and state delivery of different components of the public health-care system. However, the US represents a more starkly bipolar case, combining both highly centralized and highly decentralized programs. Medicare, the largest public program, is a purely federal program, with few intergovernmental aspects. It covers virtually all people over age 65 and about five million disabled individuals under age 65; and it represents about two-thirds of the total public health-care expenditures in the country. Policies concerning Medicare are determined by the federal Congress and the program is administered across the country by a federal agency. Throughout its life, Medicare has been sustained by strong public support, powerful bureaucratic champions, and protective congressional committees. As a result, this largest pillar of the public health insurance system operates as a single program across the country as a whole.

In contrast, the second, smaller pillar of the public system operates in a decentralized fashion. Medicaid, a health program targeted mainly at the welfare poor, and the State Child Health Insurance Program, a new initiative directed at children from low-income families, are federal-state programs supported by federal conditional grants and delivered by state governments. In Medicaid, broad federal guidelines determine general eligibility and coverage standards, but leave considerable room for states to tailor their programs to local conditions and preferences. In addition, the federal administration has the authority to grant waivers from some regulations to individual states to provide for experimentation in program design. As we will see in greater detail below, the result is that state programs vary considerably in eligibility requirements, service coverage, utilization limits, provider payment policies, reliance on managed care and spending per recipient. Moreover, the State Children's Health Insurance Program provides even more flexibility than does Medicaid.

In contrast to most other federal systems, the mediation of federal-state conflicts in the United States does not flow through formal intergovernmental mechanisms. Although the courts can and do play a role, conflicts over the terms and conditions of federal support flow into national politics, with state governments bringing pressure to bear on Congress, especially the Senate where these issues tend to be resolved. Although members of the Senate normally protect the interests of their state in battles over such issues as the funding formula for federal-state programs, they are independent political agents and do not necessarily agree with or speak for the state governor and administration in matters of general health policy. Thus, in the final analysis, it is the central government that resolves intergovernmental tensions in the federal-state components of the system.

Canada

Health policy in Canada constitutes the most decentralized of the five systems examined here. Health insurance and health services generally fall within provincial jurisdiction, and the first steps toward universal health insurance took place at the provincial level, with the province of Saskatchewan playing a leading role. Unlike Australia and the United States, the federal government does not provide any significant portion of health coverage directly to citizens as a whole.[16] Federal influence has been exerted through financial transfers to provincial governments, which facilitated the extension of provincial innovations across the country as a whole and the establishment of a pan-Canadian approach to medicare during the postwar years. However, the politics of the Canadian federation ensured from the outset that the conditions attached to federal transfers were less specific than in other federations; and the shift from conditional grants to block-funding for health care in 1977 largely eliminated day-to-day federal scrutiny of specific provincial decisions.

As Antonia Maioni's chapter highlights, Canadian health care is best thought of as a series of provincial health insurance systems operating within broad federal parameters. The federal legislation, the *Canada Health Act*, specifies that provincial insurance plans receiving federal funding must reflect five principles: they must provide universal coverage; they must cover all "medically necessary" services; they must be publicly administered; coverage must be portable outside the province; and accessibility must not be limited by user fees or extra-billing by physicians, both of which are prohibited by the Act. Within these parameters, provinces shape health policy and delivery systems as they see fit. Provincial governments define the "medically necessary" services that are actually covered, and some differences have emerged across the country. Provinces also have responsibility for the delivery process, and larger organizational differences have developed here. Provinces regulate hospitals, clinics, nursing homes, and other health institutions; they negotiate fee schedules with doctors and other health professionals; they set global budgets for hospitals; and they have the final responsibility for the costs of health care. In this context, it is not surprising that provincial governments have been taking the lead in the restructuring of health-care delivery in Canada, and that — as we shall see below — there are growing differences in the governance and delivery mechanisms in the health-care sectors across the country.

The tensions between federal parameters and provincial responsibility were intensified in the 1980s and 1990s as federal contributions to provincial health budgets were cut, especially in the 1995 federal budget. At that point, what had been a long-standing intergovernmental tension flared up into a full-fledged political warfare between the two levels of government. Unfortunately, Canada had few powerful intergovernmental mechanisms to help manage the conflicts. Unlike Germany, provincial governments have no role in the federal legislature; unlike Belgium, there were no formal requirements for advance notification and consultation; and unlike Australia, there were no standing intergovernmental institutions or expert commissions to coordinate elements of the relationship. Intergovernmental negotiations in Canada operate through an informal assemblage of committees at the level of officials, ministers, and prime ministers. In the aftermath of the 1995 cuts, the federal government and all of the provinces except Quebec reached a compact known as the Social Union Framework Agreement, which provides a modest level of structure for these processes. But by the standards of several other federations, the intergovernmental structures in Canada remain weak compared to the intensity of the divisions.

The Overall Patterns

It is striking that in all of our federations, health care operates within a broad policy framework which sets core features of the system for the country as a whole. Health care involves the provision of highly personal services to individuals in diverse settings, a circumstance that has led many theorists to suggest a decentralized approach, and the state/provincial level has important roles in all of these countries. Even in the most centralized of the five federations examined here, the federated units have some responsibilities for health institutions such as hospitals and clinics. But in none of our federations is health policy a purely regional responsibility.[17] This is true for other federations not examined in detail here, such as Switzerland, often considered one of the most decentralized systems of governance.[18]

Nevertheless, as we have seen, federations clearly differ considerably in both the comprehensiveness of the federal framework, and in the ways in which decisions about that framework are made. Setting policy parameters is a highly centralized and corporatist process in Belgium and Germany, although program management and delivery proceeds on a decentralized basis through networks of social funds. Australia and the United States are middle-level cases. In both countries, the central government has full responsibility for important components of health-care insurance, delivering the program directly to citizens. Both countries rely on shared-cost programming for other components of the system; but Australia establishes more complex conditionality for its transfers in such programs, and the state governments are more directly represented in the process of defining health policy than in the United States. Finally, Canada is the case among these five in which the common framework is most limited. The federal government delivers no significant component of the health-care system directly to citizens, and the principles associated with the Canada

Health and Social Transfer (CHST) are quite general, leaving most of the big policy decisions to provincial governments.[19]

The balance between central and regional governments is constantly evolving in federations. Pressures for further decentralization exist in virtually all of these countries, and decentralist steps have been taken in some places. However, the trend is not uniform. In some cases, pressures for cost containment, which are discussed more fully below, are generating centralizing dynamics. Germany is one country in which federal legislation has intervened more extensively than in the past in efforts to contain health expenditures. Australia also settled into a more centralized model, after brief experiments with greater decentralization in the 1980s. In other cases, pressures for decentralization have had limited impact. In Canada, the federal government's financial contribution dropped during the 1980s and 1990s, arguably weakening the political legitimacy of its role in the system. However, the policy parameters embedded in the *Canada Health Act* were not relaxed, and the federal government has recently reinstated financial contributions cut in the mid-1990s.

Moreover, where there has been decentralization in health care, it has tended to be less extensive than in other policy sectors. In Belgium, the establishment of a federal system did see the transfer of limited responsibilities for health services to the new Community and Regional governments; but social security, including health insurance, remains highly centralized in comparison with most other important policy sectors, and recent demands for decentralization advanced by the Flemish Community have been blocked. In a similar vein, the federal government in Canada accepted significant decentralization in social assistance and labour market programs, but has resisted pressures for a similar shift in health care. The decision in the United States to decentralize significant control over Medicaid is therefore something of an exception in these five countries. Even here, however, it is worth noting that although social assistance was shifted to a block-grant mechanism, a similar proposal for Medicaid was vetoed by President Clinton. In many ways, therefore, the continued role of central governments is a striking pattern in these countries. Health care seems to retain a special political sensitivity that constrains pressures for decentralization.

THE IMPACT OF FEDERALISM ON HEALTH-CARE POLICY

What then is the impact of these differences in federal institutions on health-care policy? The case studies in this volume give very different answers to this question. At one extreme, analysts from countries with powerful central frameworks and consensual decision processes tend to assign the importance of federalism to a secondary status. Johan de Cock concludes that "the impact of federal state structures on health policy (in Belgium) is still quite limited;" and Dietmar Wassener argues that "federalism will continue to play a secondary role in shaping German health care."[20] At the other extreme, Antonia Maioni concludes her study of Canada by noting that "federalism is a defining feature of the Canadian health-care model."[21] Not surprisingly, judgements about the two intermediate cases, Australia and the United States, are more qualified, and tend to focus less on the implications of federalism for the basic characteristics of health programs and more on the efficient management of the system. In Australia, Linda Hancock points to federal obstacles to efficiency and reform, citing a recent commission report that recommended "where practicable, it is best to avoid multiple levels of government involvement in the first place."[22] In the case of the United States, David Colby is similarly restrained about the importance of federalism, arguing that "our lack of rationality in program development does not lie in our federal system, but in our party system and government."[23]

A closer comparison of the experiences revealed in the country chapters, however, does throw a slightly sharper light on the influence of federal institutions on health policy. This chapter draws out those comparisons by exploring two distinct agendas that in combination define health-care politics in OECD nations: access to health care on one side, and budgetary planning on the other. In addressing the access agenda in a federal context, we concentrate on the extent to which citizens in all regions of a country receive comparable levels of health services. In addressing the planning agenda, we explore the capacity of these five countries to pursue strategies to constrain the growth of health-care expenditures.

Access to Health Care: Social Citizenship and Regional Diversity

Every federal state must establish a balance between two social values: a commitment to social citizenship, to be achieved through a common set of public services for all citizens across the entire country; and respect for regional communities and cultures, to be achieved through decentralized decision-making and significant scope for diversity in public services at the state/provincial level. The debate over this balance is an ongoing one in all federations. The discourse varies from one country to another, and in practice discussion can quickly become embroiled in amazingly technical issues of intergovernmental finance and complex points of constitutional interpretation. But the underlying question is both simple and profound. Which community should be paramount in the definition of social benefits: the community of all citizens on one hand; or regional communities defined by state/provincial boundaries on the other? There is no single answer to this question. The appropriate response will vary from federation to federation, depending on the nature of political identities and the conceptions of community embedded in its culture.

As used in this context, the concept of social citizenship is not restricted to universal programs provided to each and every citizen. Selective or targeted programs are also relevant if they function similarly across the country. The issue is whether citizens in similar economic and social situations are treated equally, irrespective of where they live in the country. Does a sick baby in one region have access to the same level of care on similar terms and conditions as a sick baby in another region of the same country? Or do the public benefits to which a citizen is entitled also depend significantly on the region in which he/she resides?

The balance between common benefits and regional diversity in federations is influenced by two key instruments: the strength of the federal policy framework established for health policy, and the strength of interregional financial transfers. As noted in the previous section, a common framework can be established in two ways. In some federations, important health programs are designed and delivered directly to citizens by the federal government, as in the case of Medicare in the United States and the Medical Benefits and Pharmaceutical Benefits schemes in Australia. These programs operate on a country-wide basis, providing all citizens with common benefits for an important component of the health-care system. A second approach is central legislation that sets policy parameters within which other agencies design and deliver health programs. In Belgium and Germany, such legislation sets the framework for social funds which administer health insurance. In other federations, federal legislation establishes parameters for state/provincial governments, as in the case of Medicaid in the United States, hospital services in Australia, and health care generally in Canada.

The second instrument critical to the agenda of social citizenship is interregional transfers. The case for a powerful system of interregional transfers in a federation lies in the conviction that citizens in all parts of a country should be entitled to comparable benefits and services without having to pay significantly different taxes.[24] Richer regions in any country enjoy the virtuous circle of fewer social needs and greater revenue capacity; poorer regions confront a vicious circle of greater social needs and weaker revenue capacity. Sustaining a common or even comparable benefit/tax regime in such circumstances inevitably requires some form of interregional transfer. Such transfers also allow federations to minimize the danger that regional differences in tax and benefit levels will begin to influence migration of both capital and individuals across the country, helping to avoid the much discussed twin dangers of "capital flight" and "welfare magnets."

In federal states, interregional transfers take two forms. In programs delivered directly by the central government, the transfers are implicit rather than explicit, resulting from the differential impact of common benefits and taxes across regions of uneven economic strength. Such transfers tend to be hidden, but they are no less real for their opaque nature. In the case of programs delivered by other authorities, whether social funds or state/provincial governments, transfers are more explicit. In Germany, health insurance is funded through contributions levied by the social funds themselves, and reducing variation in the benefit/contribution package across plans has led to the development of a major inter-fund redistribution scheme, known as the risk equalization mechanism (REM), which is well analyzed in the chapter by Wassener. Although the REM was not designed as an explicitly interregional transfer mechanism, it does have the effect of shifting resources among regions of the country. In addition, massive transfers from west Germany to east Germany have been required to create comparable standards in public services, including health care, across the old divide.

In countries in which major health programs are delivered by state/provincial governments, net interregional transfers are embedded in formal transfer mechanisms. In some cases, as occurs in a limited way in the case of Medicaid in the United States, redistribution is built into the funding formula for the program. In other countries, interregional redistribution flows through a separate program, as in the Belgian "national solidarity" grant, the Canadian equalization program, the inter-Länder transfers in Germany, and the system of adjustments to intergovernmental transfers in Australia.

The politics of interregional transfers are becoming increasingly controversial in virtually all federal states, as the various chapters in this book make clear. Interestingly, the form of redistribution does not seem to affect the intensity of political debate. One might expect the less visible, implicit transfers embedded in centrally delivered programs to be less politically contested; and certainly few people seem to care, for example, about the interregional transfers embedded in the Pharmaceuticals Scheme in Australia. However, the insulating effects of implicitness are hardly perfect. In the United States, the formula governing payments for health maintenance organizations (HMOs) under Medicare sparked a political battle between the rural and urban states, which the Senate had to resolve. More dramatically, Flemish nationalists in Belgium have mounted a powerful political challenge to the transfers implicit in the federal government's social security and health insurance programs. In this case, the opaque nature of the transfers probably created more opportunities for radical nationalist politicians to make inflammatory statements about their size.[25]

Explicit transfers to other governments or social funds can also attract political heat. Once again, however, there appears to be no neat correlation between the form of transfer and the level of controversy. Embedding interregional redistribution in the general funding formula for health programs was received with relative calm in the case of Medicaid in the United States, perhaps because no separate equalization program exists in that country.[26] In Canada, however, richer provinces traditionally fight hard against a differential formula in the federal transfer for health care, insisting that interregional redistribution should be limited to the separate equalization program. In Germany, both forms of transfer have generated recent challenges. In many ways, the commitment to interregional solidarity is strongest in Germany, and the Basic Law empowers the federal government to act to ensure "the establishment of equal living conditions throughout the federal territory."[27] Despite this commitment, political challenges have emerged in recent years. The risk equalization mechanism, which is strictly speaking an inter-fund transfer rather than an inter-Länder transfer, has been challenged legally by some health funds and politically by some Länder governments.[28] In addition, the richer Länder in the south have launched legal challenges to the general-purpose, tax-financed inter-Länder transfer scheme, complaining about the recipient regions in the north.

In the end, the politics of interregional redistribution seem rooted less in the form of the transfer, and more in the underlying level of political support for notions of solidarity and social citizenship. Federal countries differ in their tolerance of regional variations in tax and benefit packages, reflecting different levels of commitment to the equality of individual citizens on the one hand and respect for cultural differences, regional autonomy, and decentralization on the other.[29] Among our five federations, the strongest levels of interregional redistribution to support health care seem to be found in Belgium, Germany, and Australia. Canada seems to fall into an intermediate category. The Canadian constitution includes a commitment to an equalization program to support less affluent regions, but the funding formula is not as powerful as in these other federations. It is the United States, however, that defines the other end of the spectrum. There is no separate program for equalizing the fiscal capacity of state governments, and states receive relatively limited fiscal assistance from the central government, constraining the capacity of poorer states to provide average levels of public services or to introduce innovative programs on their own.[30]

In combination, the specificity of the central framework and the strength of interregional redistribution set the structural underpinnings of the balance between social citizenship and regional diversity in the definition of health care. The patterns across the five federations are summarized in Figure 2. Belgium, Germany, and Australia comprise one group, characterized by strong common frameworks and strong interregional redistribution. The United States and Canada represent contrasting cases. The United States has an intermediate framework but a low level of interregional redistribution, whereas Canada has the leanest common framework but a middle level of interregional redistribution.

These structures define the real policy room available for distinctive regional or local approaches to health care. How that policy room is used in practice depends on a much wider range of factors: the extent of cultural and political differences across the country; differences in the relative strength of stakeholders; and so on. A fuller analysis of the determinants of health-policy

FIGURE 2

Interregional Variation in Health Care: Instruments and Outcomes

Country	Instruments		Outcomes
	Specificity of Policy Framework	*Interregional Transfers*	*Interregional Differences in Health-Care Systems*
Belgium	high	high	low
Germany	high	high	low
Australia	high	high	low
United States	medium	low	medium
Canada	low	medium	medium

choices at the regional level goes beyond the scope of this study. However, the case studies in this volume do shed light on the extent of regional variation in health benefits that does result from the interaction of national frameworks, interregional redistribution, and distinctive regional societies.

Figure 2 summarizes the pattern in each of our five federations. Not surprisingly, a common standard of health benefits across the country seems strongest in Belgium, Germany, and Australia. In the case of Australia, for example, there are no significant regional variations (except for the case of the Northern Territories) in such dimensions as the number of hospital beds per 1,000 population or per capita use of medical services, and the primary geographic inequalities in access to health services tend to be between urban and rural areas within each region.[31] Moreover, the basic structure of health-care policy and delivery has become more uniform across the country with the expansion of the federal role under Medicare after 1984.

> Fifteen years ago, there were substantial differences between states in hospitalization rates, costs and public expenditures.... Most of these have disappeared. The high spending states have all pared health outlays at the same time that previously low spending ones have raised them. There were equally large structural differences within state systems. Queensland and Tasmania were traditionally "public" states, Victoria a "private" one with New South Wales having the most complex interweaving of the two. Much of this has also gone. Membership of private insurance reflected the same systemic diversity.... There is now no significant difference in coverage between the states and it would be very surprising if there were one.[32]

The impact of differences in the strength of common frameworks and interregional transfers is also highlighted by the contrast with Canada and the United States. The Canadian package of federal principles embedded in the *Canada Health Act* and equalization between rich and poor provinces produces a common approach to eligibility and a relatively common package of health services for Canadians across the country, as the tables reported in Antonia Maioni's chapter indicate. Health expenditures in poorer provinces represent a significantly higher proportion of provincial GDP than in richer provinces, something that would be highly unlikely without interregional transfers. Within these common parameters, however, the Canadian system leaves considerable scope for provincial variation; and different provincial approaches to restructuring and expenditure restraint are generating progressively larger differences in governance, management, and health service delivery. As a team of leading commentators remarked, "With the exception perhaps of Quebec, over the past twenty-five years the provincial health care systems have shared not only the five principles of Medicare but also similar delivery and management structures. In the coming years they may resemble each other only in sharing the principles of Medicare.... These divergent paths will challenge the concept of a "national" system, if such a conception ever existed."[33]

As we have seen, the US represents a bipolar case. Medicare establishes a common approach to public health services for elderly and disabled Americans, but the combination of a weak framework and weak interregional transfers in the area of health care for poor children and families means that their protections are subject to marked regional disparities. In 1994, even before welfare reform, differences in eligibility meant that Medicaid beneficiaries, as a proportion of the low-income population, varied from a high of 79 percent in Vermont to lows of 30 percent in Nevada, 36 percent in South Dakota, and 39 percent in Florida.[34] Variation in service levels are also clearly implicit in the differences in average payments per recipient of Medicaid services, which in 1998 ranged from $8,961 in New York to $2,386 in California, a difference that cannot be explained away simply as a reflection of different health costs in these two affluent states.[35]

Federalism and Access to Health Care: The Overall Pattern

The strength of the commitment to comparable access to health services is a striking feature of these federations. Despite the underlying importance of diversity embedded in the logic of federalism, these five federations have organized themselves so as to constrain interregional variation in the access to public health services enjoyed by citizens across the country. This is true both of multi-nation federations such as Belgium and Canada and federations such as Australia and Germany in which cultural diversity is less regionally concentrated. There are undoubtedly important regional variations in many federations, as evidenced by state differences in Medicaid in the United States and the increasingly distinctive delivery systems across Canada. Nevertheless, on this dimension, federal states tend to resemble non-federal ones, in which inequalities are less marked across regions than between urban and rural areas within regions. It would appear that there is limited scope for highly visible interregional differences in health services in contemporary federal systems, an issue to which we return at the end.

Cost Containment in Federal States

Federal states appear less successful in the area of fiscal restraint. Health-care systems throughout the OECD world have been under cost pressures during the last 20 years, and governments have debated a wide array of policy instruments they hope will slow the seemingly relentless growth of health expenditures. The choices have ranged from relatively blunt instruments such as global caps on expenditures for particular programs, to changes in the mix of services provided, to more complex instruments designed to change the incentives facing citizens and service providers.[36]

The approach to cost containment adopted in any individual country is shaped by the structure of its health-care system. As Tuohy has argued, the basic structure of a health-care system creates its own internal logic, which governs the way in which it responds to external pressures.[37] The structure also determines the sorts of levers that governments can hope to use most readily to constrain expenditures: the single-payer system in Canada presents different levers than the public/private mix in the United States. Changing the structure of a health-care system and creating completely new levers requires the mobilization of substantial political will by government leaders. Such major interventions are rare. The attempt by the Thatcher government in the UK to introduce "internal markets" in the National Health Service and the reform effort of the Clinton administration in the US represented two such initiatives, and both fell short of their champions' initial aspirations, dramatically so in the case of Clinton's proposed reforms. In the main, therefore, governments tend to rely on the mechanisms that the health-care system makes available to them.

Federal institutions do add an additional layer of complexity to cost containment, and it is striking that federal states seem to have greater difficulties in containing cost pressures. As Figure 3 indicates, federal states consistently devoted a larger portion of their GDP to health expenditures than did non-federal states throughout the 1960–98 period (9.9 percent versus 7.8 percent in 1998). This is true whether or not the United States, which has committed a larger portion of its GDP to health than any other OECD country since 1970, is included; excluding the United States only lowers the average for federal states in 1998 to 9.3 percent. As the more detailed data in Table A2 indicate, the rate of increase in health expenditures as a percent of GDP has also been somewhat higher in federal states than in non-federal states, a pattern

FIGURE 3

Total Health Expenditures as Percent of GDP, Federal and Non-Federal States, 1960–1998

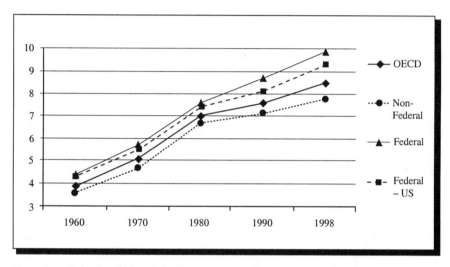

Notes: For Federal and Non-Federal, see notes to Table 1. German data in 1990s include east Germany.

Source: OECD, *OECD Health Data 2000.*

that began in the 1980s and continued into the 1990s. While health costs in federal states increased by an average of 30.3 percent between 1980 and 1998 (25.7 percent when the United States is excluded), the average increase in non-federal states was only 16.4 percent. Figure 4 indicates that the higher rate of increase also held for *public* spending on health (for more detail, see also Table A3). The increase in federal states was over 33 percent, a rate that is reduced only to about 32 percent by the exclusion of the US. Over the same time period, the increase in non-federal states was a mere 3.3 percent.

Why should federal states have greater difficulty in containing cost pressures? It has often been argued that attempts to contain health spending in one area simply shift the pressures elsewhere in the system, much as when a balloon is squeezed at one end and expands at the other. Federal systems may be more prone to cost-shifting in two directions. First, as we saw earlier, the private health sector tends to play a larger role in federations, increasing the opportunities for cost-shifting between public and private funders. Second, the

FIGURE 4

Public Health Expenditure as Percent of GDP, Federal and Non-Federal States, 1960–1998

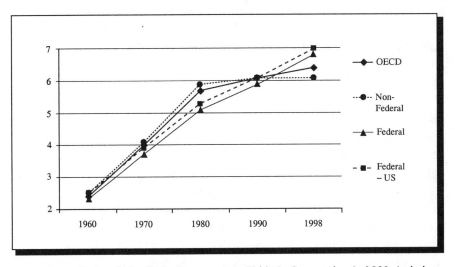

Notes: For Federal and Non-Federal, see notes to Table 1. German data in 1990s include east Germany.

Source: OECD, *OECD Health Data 2000.*

participation of two levels of government in shaping public health programs increases the chances that cost containment will involve cost-shifting between governments. The simplest form of this dynamic occurs when a central government reduces its transfers to state or provincial governments, without simultaneously easing conditions attached to the funding, as in the case of unfunded federal mandates in the United States, or the practice of the Canadian government of reducing its transfers to provinces while continuing to enforce the principles established in the *Canada Health Act.*

This logic would seem to suggest that efforts to constrain public health spending in federations will be easiest when control over the key policy instruments is effectively lodged at one level of government, whether at the federal or the state/provincial level. In cases when control over the key levels of cost containment is divided, the prospects for cost containment would seem to depend heavily on the effectiveness of mechanisms of intergovernmental coordination.

These dynamics can be illustrated by an examination of several of the countries considered in this study. As de Cock notes in his chapter on Belgium, the concentration of control over the fiscal levers in health policy in the central government virtually eliminates the scope for cost-shifting between levels of government. In the case of Germany, while service delivery by funds represents a very decentralized system, control over the key policy levers is concentrated at the national level, and the decision system requires a high level of intergovernmental consensus. In this context, federalism represented no barrier to the sweeping effort at cost containment in the *Structural Health Reform Act* of 1993. The legislation contained both a massive short-run effort to stabilize costs and a longer term strategy of structural reforms designed to alter the underlying dynamics within the health-care system. This strategy included significant changes in the system of hospital remuneration, a redefinition of the division of labour between general practitioners and specialists, controls on the number of doctors and their regional distribution, changes in reimbursement for drugs, greater competition among health funds for clients, and the risk-equalization mechanism designed to level the playing field on which they would compete. Although there was debate about the relative effectiveness of the various components of the 1993 legislation, it clearly represented a substantial package. Because the legislation affected the Länders' budgetary role in the hospital sector, the legislation had to be adopted in the Bundesrat as well as the lower house in parliament. As a result, it required an intergovernmental consensus as well as one between the social partners. Such approval is not automatic. In 2000, the federal government proposed another *Statutory Health Insurance Reform Act*, which included a comprehensive maximum budget, not just for specific areas, but for the system as a whole. The proposal had to be dropped in response to opposition in the Bundesrat. Nevertheless, the combination of central responsibility for framework legislation and a powerful mechanism of intergovernmental coordination has proven consistent with broad action on cost containment.

At the other end of the spectrum, the highly decentralized Canadian model also provides the capacity for powerful cost containment. Admittedly, the Canadian system provides some scope for burden-shifting, as noted above. The federal government shifted the potential risks inherent in health-cost pressures to provincial governments in the late 1970s when it moved from open-ended cost-sharing to block-funding. During the 1980s and 1990s, Ottawa transferred actual costs by reducing the block-fund transfer. In addition, the conditions attached to the federal *Canada Health Act* preclude certain options at the provincial level, especially those involving user fees and co-payments. Within those constraints, however, the provincial governments have the advantage of a single-payer model, which provides powerful levers for cost containment. Provincial governments have sought to limit their own financial obligations by capping hospital and then physician services budgets, and by closing many hospitals and restructuring others. In a single-payer system, service providers were left with nowhere to shift their costs, and they were drawn into expanded and intensified negotiations with provincial governments and with the regional structures established in most provinces.[38] This highly concentrated power proved relatively effective in containing costs. During the period between 1992 and 1997, when Canadian governments were struggling to eliminate their substantial deficits, public spending on health care declined an average of 2 percent each year. Although private health spending did grow somewhat in this period, the dominance of the public sector in core health services ensured a substantial slowing of overall health expenditures in Canada in that period. The consolidation of power at one level clearly does create the capacity for governments to squeeze the system when needed.

Federations in which spending responsibilities are more evenly divided between the two levels of government would seem to face larger challenges in ensuring that cost-containment efforts do not degenerate completely into cost-shifting. This challenge is illustrated most vividly in the United States, in which the multiplicity of payers in both the public and private sectors makes integrated cost-containment strategies impossible.

CONCLUSIONS

In keeping with other studies of the role of political institutions, the conclusions that flow from this study suggest that federal institutions on their own are never determinative. At the broadest level, federalism is clearly compatible with a wide range of health-care systems: large public roles; small public roles; corporatist systems relying on social partners to deliver benefits; systems relying on management through government agencies. On average, the public share of health spending in federations is somewhat smaller, a pattern that echoes findings in the larger literature on the welfare state. But, in general, the simple distinction between federal and non-federal systems does not take one very far. Other factors, including the clash of economic interests and political ideologies as well as the norms and values embedded in the underlying culture leave powerful imprints on the health-care systems that emerge in different countries.

Nevertheless, the structure of political institutions does have an important role in shaping the ways in which competing interests and groups engage in the struggle to shape health policy. From this perspective, federalism matters a great deal. But how it matters depends on the particular structure of federal institutions, and the ways in which they are rooted in the wider political environment. Laying bare these complex linkages between federal institutions and health policy requires careful examination of different federal countries, such as those appearing in the chapters of this book.

The broad patterns that emerge from these country comparisons are striking. First, in none of these federations is health policy a purely local responsibility. Federations vary enormously in the responsibilities of the central and regional governments in health policy, the role of regional governments in shaping the health policies of the central government, the nature of fiscal relations between the two levels of government, and the mechanisms for coordinating their programs. However, the central government plays a role in all of these systems, and decentralist pressures have had less impact on the balance between central and regional governments in this policy sector than in many others. The political sensitivity of health care seems to ensure that the politics of health policy resonate across the country as a whole, even in systems otherwise marked by highly regionalized policy-making.

Moreover, the particular structure of federal institutions and norms in each country has important implications for key features of the health-care system. As we have seen, federalism matters to at least two distinct agendas at the heart of health-care politics: the agenda of access to services and the agenda of rational planning. The division of labour between levels of government and the nature of interregional fiscal relations have powerful implications for the distribution of health services among citizens across the country as a whole. Whether a sick child in one region has access to the same level of treatment on comparable terms and conditions as a sick child at the other end of the country depends heavily on the often arcane details of federal institutions, norms, and fiscal relations. The extent to which federal states have succeeded in establishing interregional evenness in health services is striking. In this area, federal states look much like non-federal ones. In contrast, federations have a less enviable record in the politics of cost containment, an outcome that seems to reflect in part the greater opportunities for cost shifting created by complex governance systems in the public sector and the somewhat larger role of private health care in federal states.

These contrasting patterns may seem counter-intuitive. Given the literature on the politics of the welfare state, one might have expected federations to have greater difficulty in achieving interregional equity than in meeting other policy challenges. The distinctive record tracked here undoubtedly reflects a number of factors. First, democratic politics may be less tolerant of interregional inequality in health care than in other forms of inequality. "It is through the territorial units they live in," Sidney Tarrow reminds us, that citizens "organize their relations with the state, reconcile or fight out conflicts of interest, and attempt to adapt politically to wider social pressures."[39] Other dimensions of inequality are not represented as directly in political life. Second, the intense political salience of health care seems to constrain the politics of regional diversity, which leave a larger imprint on many other public programs in federations. David Cameron and Fraser Valentine have emphasized the difference between health care and disability policy in this regard: "health care, being of central and universal public concern, has a palpable impact on federalism.... Disability, on the other hand, being viewed to some extent as a 'niche concern,' yields a much more limited, lower profile policy discourse, which drastically reduces its capacity to affect the federal system."[40] In effect, health politics seem to influence federalism as much as federalism influences health politics.

The relationships between institutions and public policy can be subtle, complex and often difficult to disentangle from all of the other forces shaping the choices made by governments in democratic societies. Nevertheless, understanding these linkages remains important. Certainly in federations, the future of health policy will be shaped by the enduring interplay between political struggles on the one hand and the institutional framework within which politics are conducted on the other.

NOTES

[1]This chapter benefited from the research assistance of Vincent Melillo. We were also helped by comments from Jacob Hacker and participants in a policy seminar series at Brandeis University where an earlier version was presented in May 2001.

[2]For a study that draws on the experience of several federal states in order to anticipate the issues involved in the devolution of health services to regional authorities in Italy, see George France, ed., *Federalismo, Regionalismo e Standard Sanitari Nazionali: Quattro Paesi, Quattro Approcci* (Milano: Dott. A. Giuffrè Editore, 2001).

[3]World Health Organization, *The World Health Report 1999* (Geneva: World Health Organization, 1999).

[4]For discussions of this approach, see E. Immergut, "The Theoretical Core of the New Institutionalism," *Politics & Society* 26,1 (1998):5-34; F.W. Scharpf, "Institutions in Comparative Policy Research," *Comparative Political Studies* 33, 6/7 (2000):762-90, and *Games Real Actors Play: Actor-Centered Institutionalism in Policy Research* (Boulder: Westview Press, 1999); P. Pierson, "Increasing Returns, Path Dependence and the Study of Politics," *American Political Science Review* 94, 2 (2000):251-67; and K. Thelen and S. Steinmo, "Historical Institutionalism in Comparative Politics," in *Structuring Politics: Historical Institutionalism in Comparative Analysis*, ed. S. Steinmo, K. Thelen and F. Longstreth (Cambridge: Cambridge University Press, 1992). For applications to health policy, see J. Hacker, "The Historical Logic of National Health Insurance: Structure and Sequence in the Development of British, Canadian and U.S. Medical Policy," *Studies in American Policy Development* 12 (1998):57-130; E. Immergut, *Health Politics: Interests and Institutions in Western Europe* (Cambridge: Cambridge University Press, 1992); and A. Maioni, *Parting at the Crossroads: The Emergence of Health Insurance in the United States and Canada* (Princeton, NJ: Princeton University Press, 1998).

[5]G. Esping-Andersen, *The Three Worlds of Welfare Capitalism* (Princeton, NJ: Princeton University Press, 1990); and F. Castles, "Australia's Strategy for Coping with External Vulnerability," in *The Comparative History of Public Policy*, ed. F. Castles (Cambridge: Cambridge University Press, 1989).

[6]It is true that none of the five federations has established an integrated national health service on the British or Swedish model, in which the state directly delivers health services to citizens through medical professionals who are employed by the state and hospitals and other institutions owned by the state. Establishing such a comprehensive role for the state in a federation would be particularly challenging, and it is perhaps not surprising that these federal states rely on public insurance systems. We are indebted to Jacob Hacker for this point.

[7]This literature has long roots. For early examples, see H. Laski, "The Obsolescence of Federalism," reprinted in *The People, Politics and the Politician*, ed. A. Christensen and E. Kirkpatrick (New York: Holt 1941); and A.H. Birch, *Federalism, Finance and Social Legislation in Canada, Australia and the United States* (Oxford: Clarendon Press, 1955). For an excellent review of more recent literature, see P. Pierson, "Fragmented Welfare States: Federal Institutions and the Development of Social Policy," *Governance* 8, 4 (1995):449-78.

[8]A. Noël, "Is Decentralization Conservative?: Federalism and the Contemporary Debate on the Canadian Welfare State," in *Stretching the Federation: The Art of the State in Canada*, ed. Robert Young (Kingston: Institute of Intergovernmental Relations, Queen's University, 1999). Noël surveys a number of country studies, but does not consider the large cross-national quantitative literature on the subject.

[9]For a sampling of these studies, see E. Huber, C. Ragin and J. Stephens, "Social Democracy, Christian Democracy, Constitutional Structure and the Welfare State," *American Journal of Sociology* 99, 3 (1993):711-49; A. Hicks and J. Misra, "Political

Resources and Growth of Welfare in Affluent Capitalist Democracies, 1960-1982," *American Journal of Sociology* 99, 3 (1993): 668-710; A. Hicks and D. Swank, "Politics, Institutions and Welfare Spending in Industrialized Democracies, 1960-82," *American Political Science Review* 86, 3 (1992): 658-74; M. Crepaz, "Inclusion versus Exclusion: Political Institutions and Welfare Expenditures, *Comparative Politics* 31 (1998): 61-80; and D. Cameron, "The Expansion of the Public Economy: A Comparative Analysis," *American Political Science Review* 72 (1978):1243-61.

[10]D. Swank, "Political Institutions and Welfare State Restructuring: The Impact of Institutions on Social Policy Change in Developed Democracies," in *The New Politics of the Welfare State*, ed. P. Pierson (Oxford: Oxford University Press 2001).

[11]See Jacob Hacker, *The Divided Welfare State: The Battle over Public and Private Social Benefits in the United States* (Cambridge: Cambridge University Press, forthcoming). Hacker draws on new OECD data on net social expenditures, which include both public and private expenditures on central social programs, in assessing the impact of institutional factors on the balance between public and private action across countries.

[12]L. Brown-John, "Other Models of Federal Systems Reviewed," in *Federal-Type Solutions and European Integration*, ed. L. Brown-John (Lanham: University Press of America, 1995), p. 195.

[13]See especially R. Watts, *Comparing Federal Systems*. 2d ed. (Kingston and Montreal: Institute of Intergovernmental Relations and McGill-Queen's University Press, 1999).

[14]Belgian federalism is characterized by considerable asymmetry, and these responsibilities are managed by the Regional government in the French-speaking community.

[15]See also Fritz Scharpf, "The Joint-Decision Trap: Lessons from German Federalism and European Integration, *Public Administration* 66 (1988):239-78.

[16]The only exceptions are the direct federal responsibility for health care in the northern territories and for specific classes of people, such as Aboriginal peoples, members of the armed forces, and inmates in federal prisons.

[17]Interestingly, one of the strongest cases of decentralization may actually be in the new quasi-federal structure of the United Kingdom, where Scotland has assumed full control of health policy. See K.J. Woods, "Health Policy in Scotland 1997–2000: The Impact of Political Devolution" (Glasgow: University of Glasgow, unpublished manuscript).

[18]According to the Swiss constitution, health insurance is a federal responsibility. Under a major reform in 1996, federal health insurance legislation established a universal obligation on all residents of the country to insure themselves with one of the approximately 120 companies offering health insurance, and specified the package of services that companies must include in the basic health insurance scheme. Companies remain free to set their premiums, and differences do exist both within and among cantons. However, the federal legislation establishes a risk-equalization mechanism designed to offset skimming by companies, and the federal-cantonal

transfers compensate for the impact of insurance costs on low-income residents. On the post-1996 system, see E. Thuerl, "Some Aspects of the Reform of the Health Care Systems in Austria, Germany and Switzerland," *Health Care Analysis* 17 (1999):331-54. For fuller discussions of the pre-1996 system, see OECD, *The Reform of Health Care Systems: A Review of Seventeen OECD Countries* (Paris: OECD, 1994), ch. 20; and P. Lehmann, F. Gutzwiller and J. Martin, "The Swiss Health Care System: The Paradox of Ungovernability and Efficacy," in *Success and Crisis in National Health Care Systems*, ed. M. Field (New York: Routledge 1989).

[19]For a different ranking of the extent of decentralization in the health-care sector in federal states, see P.G. Forest and K. Bergeron, "Les politiques de réforme du système de santé dans cinq fédérations: une analyse de travaux scientifiques récents,"in *Federalism and Sub-National Policies*, ed. L. Imbeau (forthcoming). In assessing the level of decentralization, Forest and Bergeron appear to focus primarily on federal-state programs, and give much less attention to programs delivered directly by central governments across the country as a whole. This has substantial implications. In the case of the United States, for example, they focus on Medicaid and seem to ignore Medicare. This leads to the conclusion that health care is more decentralized in the United States than in Canada. However, this assessment seems to miss most of the public action in health care in the United States.

[20]J. de Cock, "Federalism and the Belgian Health are System," in this volume; D. Wassener, "The German Health-Care System," in this volume.

[21]A. Maioni, "Federalism and Health Care in Canada" in this volume. In a similar vein, Jacob Hacker concludes in his comparative study that "the most distinctive aspect of the Canadian welfare state ... is the prominent role that federalism has played in its development." Hacker, "The Historical Logic of National Health Insurance," p. 96.

[22]L. Hancock, "Australian Intergovernmental Relations and Health," in this volume.

[23]D. Colby, "Federal-State Relations in United States Health Policy," in this volume.

[24]Watts, *Comparing Federal Systems*, p. 50.

[25]For details, see K. Banting, "Social Citizenship and the Multicultural Welfare State," in *Citizenship, Diversity and Pluralism: Canadian and Comparative Perspectives*, ed. A.C. Cairns, J.C. Courtney, P. MacKinnon, H.J. Michelamnn and D. Smith (Montreal and Kingston: McGill-Queen's University Press, 1999).

[26]In contrast, the uneven impact on different states of the financial formula associated with the shift to block-funding in social welfare did generate intense controversy in Congress.

[27]Article 72.2 of the Basic Law for the Federal Republic of Germany. The Basic Law had originally authorized action to preserve "the uniformity of living conditions," but was recently amended to provide somewhat more flexibility in the expectations implicit in the constitutional language.

[28]We are indebted to Deitmar Wassener for this supplementary information.

[29]See Watts, *Comparing Federal Systems*, pp. 50-53.

[30]The ranking of the strength of interregional redistribution in different federations is consistent with the analyses to be found in Watts, *Comparing Federal Systems*; R. Bird, *Federal Finance in Comparative Perspective* (Toronto: Canadian Tax Foundation, 1986); and L.S. Wilson, "Lessons for Canada from Other Federal Systems," in *Equalization: Its Contribution to Canada's Economic and Fiscal Progress*, ed. R. Boadway and P. Hobson (Kingston: John Deutsch Institute for the Study of Economic Policy, Queen's University, 1998).

[31]See the data in Australian Institute of Health and Welfare, *Australia's Health 2000: The Seventeenth Biennial Health Report of the Australian Institute of Health and Welfare* (Canberra: Australian Institute of Health and Welfare, 2000), such as Tables 5.22, S30, S31 and S50. With the exception of the Northern Territory, variation on most dimensions tends to be less than +/- 10 percent of the national average. The report gives far more attention to the urban/rural divide than to inter-state differences.

[32]J. Debble, as quoted in G. Gray, "Access to Medical Care under Strain: New Pressures in Canada and Australia," *Journal of Health Politics and Law* 23, 6 (1998):905-47.

[33]J. Hurley, J. Lomas, and V. Bhatia, "When Tinkering is Not Enough: Provincial Reform to Manage Health Care Resources," *Canadian Public Administration* 37, 3 (1994):514. The authors anticipate that greater provincial variation in management and delivery will inevitably generate challenges to the basic principles of medicare as well.

[34]D. Liska and A. Salganicoff, *Medicaid Expenditures and Beneficiaries: National and State Profiles and Trends, 1988-1994*, 2d ed. Report of the Kaiser Commission on the Future of Medicaid, November 1996, Table 6. See also M. Sparer, *Medicaid and the Limits of State Health Reform* (Philadelphia: Temple University Press, 1996).

[35]US Department of Health and Human Services, Health Care Financing Administration, *A Profile of Medicaid: Chart Book 2000* (Washington, DC: Government Printing Office, 2001), Figure 2.8.

[36]For a sophisticated comparative study of the complex factors driving health costs, see OECD, *New Directions in Health Care Policy* (Paris: OECD, 1995).

[37]C. Hughes Tuohy, *Accidental Logics: The Dynamics of Change in the Health Care Arena in the United States, Britain, and Canada* (New York: Oxford University Press, 1999).

[38]Ibid., p. 249.

[39]Sidney Tarrow, "Introduction," in *Territorial Politics in Industrial Nations*, ed. Sidney Tarrow, Peter J. Katzenstein and Luigi Granziano (New York: Praeger, 1978), p. 1

[40]D. Cameron and F. Valentine, "Comparing Policy-Making in Federal Systems: The Case of Disability Policy and Programs – An Introduction," in *Disability and Federalism: Comparing Different Approaches to Full Participation,* ed. D. Cameron and F. Valentine (Montreal and Kingston: School of Policy Studies, Queen's University and McGill-Queen's University Press, 2001), p. 3.

APPENDIX

TABLE A1
Public Expenditure as Percent of Total Health Expenditures, Federal and Non-Federal States, 1960–1998

	1960	1970	1980	1990	1998	% Change				
						1960–70	1970–80	1980–90	1990–98	1960–98
Australia	47.6	67.4	62.5	67.4	69.3	42	-7	8	3	46
Belgium	61.6	87	83.4	88.9	89.7	41	-1	7	1	46
Canada	42.7	70.2	75.6	74.6	69.6	64	8	-1	-7	63
Germany	66.1	72.8	78.7	76.2	74.6	10	8	-3	-2	13
United States	23.3	36.4	41.2	39.6	44.7	56	13	-4	13	92
Average	48.3	66.8	68.3	69.3	69.6	38	2	1	0	44
OECD										
OECD	64.2*	75.2*	78.3	77.3	76.2	17	4	-1	-1	19
Non-Federal	71.2*	80.7*	83.3	81.0	79.1	13	3	-3	-2	11
Federal	53.2	65.8	68.3	69.8	70.3	24	4	2	1	32
Federal-US	58.2	70.7	72.8	74.8	74.6	21	3	3	0	28
Ratios										
Fed./Non-Fed.	0.75	0.82	0.82	0.86	0.89					
(Fed.-US)/Non-Fed.	0.82	0.88	0.87	0.92	0.94					

Notes: *Data not available for all countries. OECD Federal and OECD Non-Federal are as in Notes to Table 1. German data in 1990s include east Germany.

Source: OECD, *OECD Health Data 2000*.

TABLE A2
Total Health Expenditures as Percent of GDP, Federal and Non-Federal States, 1960–1998

| | 1960 | 1970 | 1980 | 1990 | 1998 | % Change | | | | |
						1960–70	1970–80	1980–90	1990–98	1960–98
Australia	4.7	5.4	7.0	7.9	8.5	15	30	13	8	81
Belgium	3.4	4.1	6.4	7.4	8.8	21	56	16	19	159
Canada	5.4	7.0	7.2	9.2	9.5	3	30	28	3	76
Germany	4.8	6.3	8.8	8.7	10.6	31	40	–1	22	121
United States	5.1	7.1	8.9	12.4	13.6	39	25	39	10	167
Average	4.7	6	7.7	9.1	10.2	28	28	18	12	123
OECD										
OECD	3.9	5.1	7.0	7.6	8.5	31	37	9	12	118
Non-Federal	3.6	4.7	6.7	7.1	7.8	31	43	6	10	116
Federal	4.4	5.7	7.6	8.7	9.9	30	33	14	14	125
Federal–US	4.3	5.5	7.4	8.1	9.3	28	35	9	15	116
Ratios										
Fed./Non-Fed.	1.22	1.21	1.13	1.22	1.27					
Fed.–US/Non-Fed.	1.19	1.17	1.1	1.14	1.19					

Notes: OECD Federal and OECD Non-Federal are as in the notes to Table 1. See also Notes to Table A1 for treatment of Germany.

Source: OECD, *OECD Health Data 2000*.

TABLE A3
Public Health Expenditures as a Percent of GDP, Federal and Non-Federal States, 1960–1998

	1960	1970	1980	1990	1998	% Change			
						1960–70	1970–80	1980–90	1990–98
Australia	2.2	3.6	4.4	5.3	5.9	64	22	20	11
Belgium	2.1	3.6	5.3	6.6	7.9	71	47	24	20
Canada	2.3	4.9	5.4	6.9	6.6	113	10	28	-4
Germany	3.2	4.6	6.9	6.6	7.9	44	50	-4	20
United States	1.2	2.6	3.7	4.9	6.1	120	42	32	24
Average	2.2	3.9	5.1	6.1	6.9	77	31	19	13
OECD									
OECD	2.4	4	5.7	6.1	6.4	63	42	7	5
Non-Federal	2.5	4.1	5.9	6.1	6.1	64	44	3	0
Federal	2.3	3.7	5.1	5.9	6.8	61	38	16	15
Federal–US	2.5	3.9	5.3	6.1	7.0	56	36	15	15
Ratios									
Fed./Non-Fed.	0.92	0.9	0.86	0.97	1.11				
Fed.–US/Non-Fed.	1.00	0.95	0.9	1.00	1.15				

Notes: For OECD Federal and OECD Non-Federal, see Notes to Table 1. For treatment of Germany, see Notes to Table A1.

Source: Calculated from *OECD Health Data 2000*.

2

FEDERALISM AND THE BELGIAN HEALTH-CARE SYSTEM

Johan de Cock

INTRODUCTION

Belgium provides a fascinating perspective on the complex interplay among cultural diversity, federal institutions, and public policy outcomes. Created originally as a unitary state, Belgium has gradually been transformed into a federation over the last 30 years. Constitutional decentralization was sought primarily for cultural and linguistic reasons, and not because public policy necessarily required a more decentralized approach. Nevertheless, the impact of the "federalization" of the state on the way public policy is carried out in a number of sectors, such as education and economic policy, is substantial. Health-care policy remains largely in the hands of the federal government, and has been less affected so far. However, even here, intergovernmental coordination has become much more important. In addition, calls for the federalization of health care have now become commonplace in Flemish political circles, and the constitutional future of the sector is very much in contention. This chapter seeks to describe the Belgian health-care system, to analyze the impact of the country's newly federal institutions on health-care policy, and to shed light on the current debate concerning its potential devolution.

THE BELGIAN FEDERATION

Belgian society is composed of two main language groups: the Dutch-speaking Flemish group, which represents about 60 percent of the population, and the French-speaking Walloon group, which represents close to 40 percent. (There is also a very small German-speaking community in the southeast of the country.) This linguistic divide has recently been translated into a decentralized constitutional system, as Belgium has gradually been transformed from a unitary to a federal state over the last 30 years. The basic federalization process occurred over four successive stages of institutional reform (1970, 1980, 1989, 1993), and it was not until the year 1994 that the country was described officially as "federal." Reaching this threshold did not complete the process, however, and another phase of constitutional reform was triggered in 2001. During this federalization process, constitutional powers have been increasingly devolved to two new, distinct sets of subnational entities — Communities and Regions. It is the co-existence of these two overlapping types of structures that make governance in Belgium both complex and unique.

Belgium is divided into three Regions: the Dutch-speaking Flemish Region in the north, the French-speaking Walloon Region in the south, and the bilingual Brussels-Capital Region. The last region has a predominantly francophone population, but is an enclave in the Dutch-speaking Flemish Region. The division into Regions was a response to the francophones' wish for greater socio-economic autonomy, and the regional governments mainly have jurisdiction over economic and land-based matters.

Belgium is also divided into three cultural Communities: the Dutch-speaking Flemish Community, with jurisdiction in Flanders and the Dutch-language institutions in Brussels; the French Community, with jurisdiction in the French-speaking south of the country and the French language institutions in Brussels; and a German-speaking Community, serving the 65,000 German-speakers in the southeast of the country. The division into Communities was a response to the Flemish wish to provide cultural autonomy for the different linguistic groups in Belgium. A purely territorial division, such as the regional one, was not possible because the Flemish authorities wished to maintain a very active presence in Brussels, an historically Flemish city that became dominated by the French in the nineteenth century. The Communities enjoy constitutional powers in relation to education and culture and various forms of "assistance to persons" for which the language used by public authorities was considered particularly important.

Several distinctive features of Belgian federalism stand out here. First, it is centrifugal: it arose from the decentralization of a unitary state rather than the voluntary alliance of previously sovereign units.[1] This trend marks all public policy debates including, as we shall see, debates over the organization of health care. Second, Belgian federalism is bipolar: although it consists of three Regions and three Communities, the logic behind the structure of the state is governed by the reality of two major language groups. The successive constitutional reforms were introduced in response to conflict and differences of opinion between these groups, and many important federal institutions are parity-based, giving equal weight to Dutch- and French-speakers in decision-making. Third, the Belgian federal system also allows for a substantial degree of asymmetry. While powers are devolved in the same fashion to similar entities, the federated entities are free to organize their institutions differently. The most striking example of this asymmetry is the merger of the Flemish Community and Regional institutions (discussed in more detail below), which has not been duplicated in the French part of the country.

The Institutions of Belgian Federalism

Belgium has developed a complex set of political institutions to give political life to its newly federal nature. The federal Parliament, which is elected every four years, is bicameral, with a House of Representatives and a Senate. The House of Representatives has 150 members who are elected by proportional representation, and are subdivided into a French-speaking and a Dutch-speaking group. The second chamber, the Senate, has 71 members. The majority of Senators are directly elected, but a significant number are designated by, and from, the legislative assemblies of two main linguistic Communities. The Senate is thus partly the chamber of the "Communities," illustrating again the bipolar nature of the Belgian federal system. Some matters can be legislated exclusively by the House of Representatives, while others also require the concurrent intervention of the Senate.

While the composition of the federal Parliament reflects the Dutch-speaking majority, the federal Cabinet is composed of an equal number of French-speaking and Dutch-speaking ministers. The prime minister is always Flemish, but he or she is normally bilingual and is seen as "linguistically neutral" and therefore not part of the parity calculations. This norm of parity represents an important guarantee for the French-speaking minority.

In contrast to the federal Parliament, the legislatures of the Communities and Regions are unicameral. They are elected for five years, and issue "decrees" that are legally equivalent to federal legislation. As noted above, there has been a fusion between the institutions of the Flemish Community and Region. The Flemish Parliament has 118 seats, and the decrees that it issues in its regional role apply to the Flemish Region. When voting on decrees related to "Community" matters, however, the 118 members are joined by six Dutch-speaking members from the Brussels Regional Parliament, and these decrees apply both in the Flemish Region and in the Brussels Region on Flemish Community matters such as cultural or social institutions that function solely in Dutch.

The Walloon Parliament, which has 75 seats, issues decrees on regional matters, which are valid in the Walloon Region.[2] The francophone Community Parliament remains legally separate, but is not directly elected. It is composed of all 75 members of the Walloon Regional Parliament, as well as 19 francophone members of the Brussels Regional Parliament, and its decrees on Community matters are valid in the Walloon Region and in the Brussels Region.

As complex as these institutions may seem, the arrangements in Brussels are even more so. The 75 members of the Brussels Regional Parliament are elected on unilingual lists. At present, there are 64 French-speaking members and 11 Dutch-speaking members, which corresponds more or less to the estimated language split in the Brussels Region. This Parliament issues "ordinances"[3] on regional matters, which apply in the Brussels Region. The government is composed of a "minister-president," whose election requires a majority of both language groups in the Parliament, and two French-speaking and two Dutch-speaking ministers who need the support of the majority of their respective language groups. This parity is the mirror image, in the capital, of the federal Cabinet, except that this time it offers protection to the Dutch-speaking minority in Brussels. Parliament decides on regional matters with a simple majority.

In the case of Community issues, however, the Brussels Parliamentarians sometimes sit with different hats on, for example, the Joint Community Commission deals with bilingual community matters in Brussels such as *bilingual* social services or hospitals. Decisions of this commission require a "double majority," that is, a majority in each language group. However, matters that only affect institutions working in French are subject to legislation by the French Community Commission (COCOF), which is composed of the French-speaking members of the Brussels Regional Parliament. There is no parallel for the institutions functioning in Dutch in Brussels, since the Flemish Community Commission (VGC) simply implements, in Brussels, the decrees of the Flemish Parliament. In other words, the COCOF is a legislative body, while the Flemish Community Commission is not. This is another example of formal symmetry but asymmetry in practice: the different groups had similar powers to organize their political structures, but they chose to do it differently.

The Distribution of Powers

The distribution of powers is set out in the *Constitutional Act*, as well as various "special Acts" which must be adopted by both a two-thirds overall majority in the federal Parliament and a majority in each language group. The Belgian federal system is characterized by a scheme of exclusive legislative powers. There are no concurrent powers, and therefore no rule such as federal paramountcy. The distinct legislative powers are often closely related, and a single policy field which would be subject to concurrent powers in some federations may well, in Belgium, be conceived as involving completely distinct and exclusive matters. As a result, the division of powers is defined very finely. Residual power is supposed to be transferred to the federated entities. However, because the French- and Dutch-speakers cannot agree on whether the Regions or the Communities should inherit this power, it has, up to now, remained federal. As a result, a matter that does not clearly fall within an enumerated head of power is federal by default.

The legislative powers of the three Regions (Flanders, Wallonia, and Brussels) essentially concern those issues that are territorially-based. They include: urban planning, environmental issues, rural development and conservation, housing, water policy; economic affairs (but not monetary policy, price and income policies, or social security), energy policy (with the exception of national infrastructure and nuclear energy), administrative control of municipalities, employment policy (but not labour law), public works and transport; and international cooperation and research as they pertain to these powers.

The legislative powers of the Communities (Dutch-, French-, and German-speaking) include linguistically sensitive matters: education; cultural programs such as the promotion of language, the arts, libraries, radio and television broadcasting; youth policy, leisure and tourism; "personalized" matters such as "assistance to individuals"; the use of language except in the localities with a "special status" where administrative services in the language of the minority must be available; and international cooperation and research with regards to those powers.

Through the successive stages of constitutional decentralization, the federal government has retained its jurisdiction over a limited number of important fields such as defence, justice, security, fiscal and monetary policy, and social security. The federal jurisdiction over social security is central to the organization of the welfare state in Belgium, including the health-care sector. While many aspects of the making of social policy have been transferred to the Communities and to lesser degree to the Regions, the federal government still has exclusive jurisdiction over the well-developed social security apparatus, with powerful consequences for the distribution of powers over health-care policy.

Financing the Federation

Over the last ten years, the expenditures of the federal authority and the Communities and Regions have evolved as follows:

TABLE 1
Expenditures, 1987–1999
(in billion BEF)

	Federal Authority (*)		Communities and Regions	
	Expenses	*Receipts*	*Expenses*	*Receipts*
1987	1911.0	1452.8	152.5	173.2
1997	1619.8	1444.6	1037.3	1034.7
1999 (budget)	1716.5	1569.9	1110.3	1098.6

Note: *Without social security.
Source: Data supplied by the National Sickness and Invalidity Insurance Institute, Brussels.

This table illustrates the significant increase in the expenditures of the Communities and the Regions over the last decade due largely to the 1988 transfer to the Communities of jurisdiction in the field of education. Interestingly, the federated entities enjoy very little autonomy in revenue collection, and 90 percent of the financial resources of the Communities and Regions come from transfers of portions of the income taxes and the value-added tax collected by the federal government. Communities do have the constitutional power to raise their own taxes, but have never exercised it because it would require the population of Brussels to opt formally for one or other Community. This is seen as involving the imposition of "subnationalities" on individual citizens, a prospect that has always been rejected by political leaders on both sides of the linguistic border. However, the lack of independent fiscal capacity does not significantly erode the autonomy of the Communities and Regions. Conditional grants are a rare phenomenon in Belgium, and the federated entities enjoy a significant degree of independence with regards to spending and policy choices in their own spheres of jurisdiction.

Finally, an equalization mechanism has been introduced in favour of the poorer Walloon and Brussels Regions. This redistribution instrument has come under strong criticism in Flanders and partly explains a call for increased financial autonomy and responsibility for the distinct federated entities, which is discussed more fully below.

Federalism and Political Parties

Over the last 20 years, all national political parties have split along linguistic lines. Members of the federal Parliament are elected either by the Flemish population through Dutch-speaking parties, or by the francophone population through French-speaking parties. As a result, there are no truly federal parties, and voices for the "whole of Belgium" are rare on the political scene. Governments are constituted of complex coalitions of parties from both sides of the linguistic divide. The federal government is composed of six parties: the distinct French- and Dutch-speaking versions of the Liberals, the Socialists, and the Greens.

The party system has important implications for relations between the different orders of government. Until 1993, members of the federal Parliament were also members of the legislative assemblies of the federated entities. Under this arrangement, political *concertation* between different levels was particularly strong. Since 1993, however, the direct election of Regional Parliaments has created a new dynamic as parliamentarians from different levels of government increasingly defend distinct visions of the future of their communities. Nevertheless, it is worth underlining that the same parties are active at the federal and at the Community and Regional levels.[4] As a result, differences of opinion between orders of government are still usually addressed *within* the partisan political structure. This is where policy development and the search for compromise essentially take place.

These are the complex and often unique political institutions of Belgian federalism. This new federal state was superimposed on an expansive welfare state, including a comprehensive system of health care created in an earlier era of unitary government, and sorting out the new governing relationships has been a challenging process. The next section describes the essential features of the Belgian health-care system, and the following one examines the relationships between health care and the new federal institutions.

THE BELGIAN HEALTH-CARE SYSTEM

Most health-care expenditures flow through the health and invalidity insurance scheme, which is an integral part of the federal social security system. As such, it is defined by five general principles: it is compulsory; it protects the insured person and his/her dependants against health-care costs as well as loss of income due to sickness; it combines insurance and solidarity mechanisms; it is managed jointly by "social partners" (management and labour), as well as other relevant interests, such as the *mutualities* or sickness funds; and it is primarily financed through contributions from employers and employees, although these are supplemented by federal subsidies and specific "solidarity" taxes.

The compulsory sickness insurance program, which covers the entire population, is composed of two different plans. The first plan, which covers approximately 93 percent of the population, is intended for salaried workers, civil servants, and comparable categories of employees, as well as their dependants. They are covered for all aspects of health care: ambulatory care (visits to the doctor); hospital care; medical care provided by medical specialists, dentists, nurses, paramedical care (such as physiotherapy); and pharmaceuticals. The second plan, which covers the remaining 7 percent, is intended for self-employed workers. This plan only covers "major risks," such as hospital care and special technical services, but the sickness funds offer supplementary insurance to cover "minor risks." About 70 percent of the self-employed subscribe to this plan, thereby benefiting from the same coverage as salaried workers.

Individuals must register with one of the private sickness funds or the public insurance fund. These funds or *mutualities* are non-profit organizations, and were originally founded either on ideological lines (christian, socialist, liberal) or on a professional basis. However, the ideological underpinnings of the system are no longer very clear and affiliation tends to depend on other factors, such as family history or ease of access. It is worth underlining that the sickness funds still function on a national basis, and are not divided by language. So far at least, they all function in Dutch in Flanders, in French in Wallonia, in both French and Dutch in Brussels, and in German in the German-speaking territory. There are, however, some indications of the development of distinctive "products" in the north and in the south in the area of supplementary insurance. For example, the French division of the largest sickness fund recently launched a specific hospital insurance scheme that was not introduced in Flanders.

Patients have free choice of health-care providers, including physicians and hospitals. Everybody has the right to unlimited access to health services and reimbursement; the services provided by the health-care insurance are granted at the beginning of an illness for an unlimited period, as long as the beneficiary keeps his/her insured status.

The governance of the health-care insurance system is corporatist in style. Management is lodged in two bodies of the National Sickness and Invalidity Insurance Institute (NSIII). The General Council, which deals with financial issues such as the annual budget, is composed of representatives of employers, salaried workers, sickness funds, and federal government.[5] Health-care providers attend meetings of the council, but in an advisory capacity only. However, the second body, the Insurance Committee, which deals with the actual organization of the insurance system, brings together representatives of the sickness funds and health-care providers.

Ambulatory Care

Both general practitioners (GP) and specialists are independent professionals who are paid by the fee-for-service method and usually have private practices. The patient is free to approach either a general practitioner or a specialist for a primary consultation. For some years now, there has been an attempt to differentiate the roles of GPs and specialists by designating GPs as the "primary" service and requiring patients to be referred by them to specialists. Support for this proposal is particularly strong in the Flemish side of the country, but is resisted by Flemish specialists and by the French-speaking medical profession more generally.

Services are charged according to a fee schedule established between the representatives of the medical profession and the sickness funds. The schedule must fit within the scope of a budgetary target defined by the General Council of the NSIII; and for the agreement to be implemented on a national scale, it must be approved by 60 percent of practitioners. The so-called "conventioned" practitioners must respect the fee schedule, except in some specific circumstances such as in case of admission in a single-occupancy hospital room. Those practitioners who do not accept the agreement are free to fix their own fees, but their patients are still only reimbursed according to the fee schedule provided for in the agreements. In the past few years, 15 percent of practitioners have chosen to fix higher fees, practising what Canadians would call "extra-billing."

The Belgian system includes co-payments by patients. The insured person must pay 30 percent of the fee for consultation with a GP, 35 percent for home visits, and 40 percent for the services of a specialist. There is, however, a preferential scheme for socially underprivileged groups such as widows, disabled persons, old age pensioners, orphans with low income, and persons living on social welfare. In the case of consultations with a physician or dentist, the patient must pay the full amount and is then reimbursed for the fund's share on submission of the bill. However, the third-party system is commonly used for technical services such as laboratory tests or radiology and is compulsory in the case of hospitalization. Insured persons receive the same level of reimbursement for insured services regardless of their sickness fund. Supplementary private sickness insurance to cover the patient's share of the costs, while increasing, is still not widespread.

Pharmaceuticals are covered in a similar fashion. Nearly 2,500 pharmaceutical products (out of 6,000) have been declared eligible for reimbursement, with the level of refund depending on therapeutic value. Vital drugs are totally refunded, while "essential" ones are refunded at a rate of 75 percent. Oral contraceptives receive a 20 percent refund, while "comfort" drugs are not refunded at all. To be refunded, a drug must have been prescribed by a practitioner, and physicians are free to prescribe the medication they prefer. Generic medications are not widely used, and drugs can only be delivered by a pharmacist.

Similarly, nursing care and physiotherapy delivered outside hospitals can be paid for by the health-care insurance scheme provided they have been prescribed by a physician. These services are supplied by salaried or self-employed nurses and are refunded either on a per-service basis or through a daily lump-sum payment based on the patient's level of dependency. Except for those benefiting from a preferential scheme, patients pay 25 percent of the nursing or paramedical costs, and 40 percent in the case of physiotherapy (although in practice a lower percentage is often applied).

Hospital Care

Hospital care amounts to 45 percent of the health insurance expenditures. As of 1 January 1998, there were 193 general hospitals registered in Belgium, of which 40 percent belong to the public sector (mainly Public Centre for Social Welfare at the municipal level) and 60 percent belong to the non-governmental, non-profit sector. At present, there are some 55,000 hospital beds for a population of roughly 10 million. For the last 15 years, the central government sought to reduce the number of hospital beds by converting acute-care beds into beds in nursing homes and by encouraging a concentration of hospital beds. This is done through various financial incentives and by imposing a minimum of 150 beds for accreditation.

A global budget for hospital operating costs for the entire country is established by the central government on a yearly basis. A quarter of these costs are financed by the federal Ministry of Health and the balance by the National Sickness and Invalidity Institute. The Communities provide capital costs for construction and the purchase of equipment is financed at a rate of 60 percent or 70 percent in the case of public hospitals.

While hospital operating costs are regulated by the federal Ministry of Health, the cost of health care provided by physicians and medical personnel is entirely financed by the sickness insurance plan. As for the ambulatory sector, medical and paramedical fees are fixed by agreement, which are negotiated at the federal level. As a rule, the fees of medical services are the same in the ambulatory and hospital sectors. Nevertheless, certain services are financed by a lump sum payment and not by the system of fee-for-service, especially in areas such as clinical biology and, to a lesser extent, medical scanning.

Physicians receive the full medical fees. They then remit a portion of those fees to the hospital pursuant to agreements with hospital management, in order to finance certain hospital costs (staff, premises). The method of payment varies greatly from one hospital to another and depends on the relationship between physicians and hospital managers.

A hospitalization lump sum of BEF 1,100 is charged to the patient for each separate hospital stay. In addition, there is a daily co-payment of BEF 450 for the in-patient costs and a daily co-payment of BEF 25 for medicines. For some categories of insured persons, those amounts are limited. Complementary insurance for hospitalization is becoming more and more common.

The health-care insurance scheme also pays for the cost of nursing care and the cost of assistance with daily activities in "rest and nursing homes" for

50   *Johan de Cock*

FIGURE 1
Financial Flows in Health Care

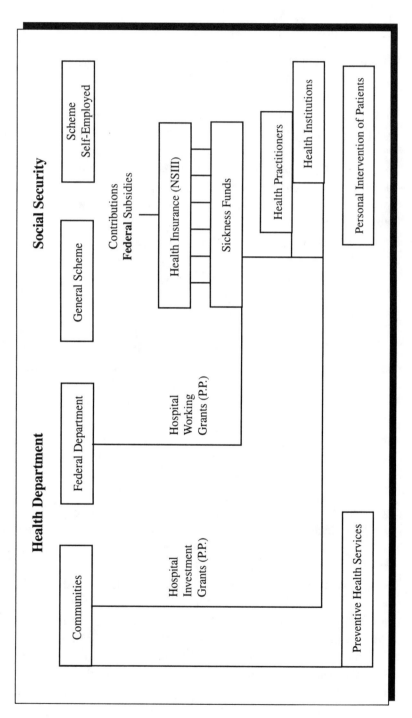

elderly people. The amount of the intervention depends on the person's level of dependency. The insured patients must pay for their own board and lodging.

Financing Health Care Insurance

OECD figures show that Belgian health expenditures amounted to 7.6 percent of gross national product (GNP) in 1996, and the complex financial flows involved are set out in Figure 1. As noted earlier, health-care insurance revenues come from ear-marked contributions by employers and employees, federal subsidies and so-called "alternative financing" composed of a special crisis tax and of a percentage of the VAT. The contribution of salaried workers is equivalent to 7.55 percent of their wages. The contribution of self-employed workers amounts to 3.84 percent of their revenues. Pensioners pay a contribution to the extent that their pension exceeds a certain ceiling.

The NSIII transfers funds to the *mutualities* on a monthly basis, in order to allow them to pay physicians and hospital bills, and to refund patients for the cost of ambulatory care. Funds are apportioned to the different sickness funds by taking into consideration a variety of risk factors such as age, sex, household composition, or the level of urbanization. Solidarity mechanisms are thus in place to ensure that no fund is disadvantaged because it caters to groups representing heavier risks than others (the elderly, industrial workers, etc.).

THE INTERACTION BETWEEN FEDERALISM AND HEALTH CARE

The meshing of a complex health-care system with new federal institutions posed important issues for Belgians, issues that are still being debated intensely.

The Distribution of Powers in Health Care

As already mentioned, the greatest part of the health-care system — the insurance scheme — is an integral part of the social security system, which so far remains under exclusive federal jurisdiction.[6] The central government also has the constitutional responsibility for fundamental aspects of health-care institutions, notably the framework legislation governing medical practice and health-care institutions such as hospitals. In 1980, the Communities were granted apparent jurisdiction over "health-care policy," resulting in a transfer of 4,735 civil servants from the federal level to the Community level.[7] Never-theless, the transfer of jurisdiction was subject to important exceptions in favour of the central state.[8] In this area, there is no doubt that the exceptions consti-tute the rule: as Table 2 indicates, 97 percent of total health-care expenditures remain in the area of federal jurisdiction. As we will see below, Flemish au-thorities have expressed dissatisfaction with the largely symbolic nature of the transfer of jurisdiction in health care.

The precise distribution of powers between the central state, Communi-ties, and Regions is complex, and differs according to the type of institution or care.[9] The federal government remains responsible for ambulatory care, the largest part of which is physician services. Health-care insurance finances the care, and federal framework legislation governs the practice of medicine, the

TABLE 2
Health Care Expenditure Per Authority, 1997

	BEF (billion)
Federal	
Federal budget	40.6
Social security–health care insurance	
Salaried workers	443.3
Self-employed workers	33.4
Subtotal	517.3 (96.5%)
Communities/Regions	
Flemish Community	9.2
French Community	5.5
Walloon Region	2.4
Brussels-Joint Community Commission	0.4
Brussels-French Community Commission	0.6
German-speaking Community	0.6
Subtotal	18.7 (3.5%)
Total	536.0(100.0%)

Source: Data supplied by the National Sickness and Invalidity Insurance Institute, Brussels.

availability of pharmaceuticals and other major aspects of health care. The Communities' responsibilities are especially limited here: they have jurisdiction over the organization and management of home care (but not for financing the care itself), and over ambulatory mental health services.

Health care in hospitals is a more complex case, although the federal role still predominates. Federal heath-care insurance finances the operating costs of hospitals, and federal framework legislation sets accreditation standards and standards concerning staff and equipment. The federal government is also responsible for the purchase of major medical equipment, standards concerning planning, and the designation of academic hospitals or services. The Communities do have responsibility in the hospital sector, but their actions in many areas are heavily constrained by federal norms and policies.[10] The Communities' basic role concerns capital investment. As mentioned earlier, they are responsible for 60 percent of the financing of hospital capital investment generally, and 70 percent in the case of public hospitals. As a result, the Communities establish priorities for hospital construction, renovations, and the purchase of equipment, including major medical equipment (although regulations concerning financing in the case of equipment remain federal). The Communities are also responsible for medical inspections and for the opening and closing of hospitals, although in both cases they must follow federal norms; and they have jurisdiction over the internal organization of hospitals but only to the extent they do not have an impact on the hospital budget. The law stipulates that Communities must communicate their decisions, including those pertaining to individual cases, to the federal government, so that federal officials can assure themselves that central norms are being respected.

In contrast to ambulatory and hospital care, the role of the Communities is dominant in health education and preventive medicine. They are responsible for providing medicine in schools, sports medicine, and occupational medicine. In the case of preventive health care, they provide information and sanitary education, and public health programs such as protection for mothers and children, the prevention of tuberculosis and cancer, and the fight against transmitted diseases. However, even preventive health care is interwoven with divided jurisdiction. For example, although vaccination is generally a Community responsibility, it is considered federal if there is a legal obligation to vaccinate, as in the case of poliomyelitis. There are also "mixed" diseases, such as hepatitis B. The federal government pays for the vaccine, but the Communities organize the vaccination campaign. On this matter, a formal cooperation agreement was signed.

Finally, the Communities also have a role in running nursing homes for the elderly. The 1980 *Institutional Reform Act* transferred jurisdiction to the Communities for so-called "personalized" matters that directly affect individuals, and for which the use of language by public authorities is deemed particularly important. Central to these personalized matters is "assistance to persons," including the financing and management of "rest" homes for the elderly. Once again, however, jurisdictions overlap. Communities are responsible for the operation of rest homes, but the medical and paramedical care offered in these institutions remains a federal matter, paid for by the national health-care insurance scheme. Not surprisingly, this division has created difficulties.

Despite these complex details, the overall distribution of powers can be summarized reasonably simply. The federal government has the leading role in the provision of health care. Although the Communities have responsibility for certain institutions, they are tightly constrained by federal legislation and their primary role is to implement federal norms. They can adopt supplementary norms, but only if they have no financial impact on the federal level. Only in the area of preventive medicine do Communities enjoy more significant powers, since they can actually legislate and regulate in this field.

The distribution of powers concerning health care has some advantages in the effort to control costs in the field of curative care. The basic instruments that have a significant impact on costs are within federal jurisdiction, especially in the three fields of ambulatory care, hospital care, and pharmaceuticals. The powers remaining with the federal government show a close connection with planning and/or financing. As a result, a well-known phenomenon in many federal systems — financial dumping by one order of government onto another — is still very modest in Belgium. The only example is the shifting of the costs of medical staff in homes for disabled children and services for preventive mental health care from the Communities to the federal level, where the health insurance program has absorbed the costs.

Mechanisms of Intergovernmental Coordination

The complicated distribution of powers in federal Belgium and the resulting need to ensure coherence between the different orders have led to complicated forms of "cooperative federalism." Maintaining sufficient collaboration and solidarity is not easy in this bipolar state, putting considerable pressure on the federal structure. In partial response to this challenge, the principle of "federal loyalty" has been constitutionalized (article 143, section 1). This principle holds that no decision of any order of government may endanger the federal construction, and each order must take into consideration the interests and the sensitivities of other orders before taking legislative action.

There are a number of other forms of cooperation, some of which are used more frequently than others in the health sector. It is worth noting that these cooperative mechanisms take place between public agents, and that the "social partners," who are central to the management of much of the welfare state, are not formally involved in these intergovernmental processes.

Mutual Representation. This mechanism involves the representation of governments on bodies that fall under the jurisdiction of another order of government. For instance, the planning commission for medical supply, which was created in 1996 by the federal Ministry of Social Affairs and Health, is composed of representatives designated by both the federal and Community levels. Another example is the Scientific Council of the National Sickness and Invalidity Institute, which is under federal jurisdiction, but can also be consulted by the Regions and Communities, to the extent they exercise jurisdiction in the field of health policy.

Obligation to Provide Information. Another mechanism is a legislated obligation to share information. For instance, the Communities must inform the federal authorities of their decisions concerning the accreditation and closing of hospitals and other health-care institutions, as well as decisions on capital investment in this sector. In March 2000, a cooperation agreement was signed in which a program of mutual data transmission is set out.

Compulsory Consultation. The *Special Institutional Reform Act* introduced different consultative procedures, ranging from the transmission of information to the conclusion of preliminary agreements. However, none of these compulsory procedures apply in the health sector.

Formal Cooperation Agreements. Another procedure is a formal cooperation agreement, to which the federal government, Communities, and Regions can be parties. Although such agreements may not modify the constitutional distribution of powers, they have legal status and cannot be modified unilaterally by the legislature of one of the signatories. Interestingly, the approval of such agreements parallels procedures established earlier for international treaties. Agreements that deal with existing legislative norms or that might put a financial burden on the federal state, the Communities, the Regions or Belgian citizens, require formal approval by the legislative assemblies of the parties to the agreement.

Cooperation agreements mostly deal with the joint creation and management of common services and institutions, the joint exercise of certain powers or the development of common initiatives. In some cases, the conclusion of cooperation agreements is compulsory; the need for them was anticipated at the time powers were devolved. In the health-care sector, there is no such legal obligation to conclude cooperation agreements. Nevertheless, several have been signed: for example, a federal government-Community agreement launched a research program into AIDS, and another established an Advisory Committee on Bioethics.

Protocols. Other agreements such as Protocols, which are less formal and do not have legal standing, are used more frequently. The Council of State[11] has noted on several occasions that even in the absence of a legal obligation to adopt formal cooperation agreements, cooperation is essential to the proper implementation of certain legislative provisions. In the health sector, draft agreements have been concluded, especially on efforts to control health costs, sometimes following the advice of the Council of State:

- measures aimed at controlling and reducing the number of beds in general hospitals;
- a timetable from 1985 to 1998 for the construction and refurbishing of hospitals or health-care institutions;
- the freezing of medical services, closing of acute beds, conversion of certain types of hospital beds, and determination of the legal status of one-day hospitalizations;
- health-care policy toward elderly people;
- the organization and financing of an inquiry on public health;
- prevention, especially vaccination against hepatitis B; and
- transmission of mutual data.

Concertation Committee and Interministerial Conferences. Finally, the *Special Institutional Reforms Act* introduced a new institution, the Concertation Committee, whose mandate is to prevent "conflict of interest" between different components of the state. This committee is composed of ministers of the different federated entities, and is chaired by the federal prime minister. It normally meets on a monthly basis, but can be called to deal with a particular crisis. The Concertation Committee can form ad hoc interministerial conferences composed of members from the executive of both orders of government in order to provide a flexible structure to coordinate policies in various matters, including health policy. Decisions taken in the framework of the conferences are not binding, but the conferences provide an important forum for drafting cooperation agreements and other forms of accord.

If conflicts cannot be settled through political processes such as interministerial conferences, or if issues of constitutionality are raised after the adoption of legislative measures, the Court of Arbitration may be apprised of the matter. The Court of Arbitration is a constitutional court with a well-defined jurisdiction. It can revoke or suspend a federal Act or a decree or ordinance of a federated entity on the grounds that it contravenes specific constitutional protections of fundamental freedoms or violates the distribution of powers. A judge in a regular court, confronted with a constitutional question can also submit it to the Court of Arbitration by means of an interlocutory question.[12] The composition of the court follows the bipolar federal model, with six Dutch-speaking and six French-speaking judges. Half of these judges are former politicians and half are professional magistrates.

The Court of Arbitration has delivered several important rulings concerning the health-care sector. For instance, the court has ruled that:

- emergency medicine, including the introduction of a single-number call system (the "100") and the obligation for physicians and hospitals to respond to calls from the service, constitutes a distinct and separate constitutional matter. In the absence of an express allocation, it falls within the federal residual power (rulings 47/95 and 63/95);
- the jurisdiction of Communities regarding health policy does not include the power to regulate medical practice (ruling 69/92);
- the federal legislature, which regulates the practice of medicine and the paramedical professions, can set conditions relating to studies and training, despite the fact that education is a Community matter. More specifically, by requiring four years of training for physiotherapy, without specifying if this training must be organized at the university or at the high school level, the federal legislature does not unduly infringe on the Communities' power over education (ruling 81/86;
- the Communities have jurisdiction over preventative medicine and health education, and consequently over anti-smoking campaigns. However, this does not include the power to prohibit tobacco advertising, because

tobacco is legally defined as a "foodstuff" which falls under federal jurisdiction (rulings 6/92, 7/93 and 17/93);

- the Communities are competent to issue decrees concerning the control of sports medicine as an integral part of preventive medicine (ruling 69/92);
- the federal legislature may introduce an external peer-review system for specific medical disciplines that affect several services and different hospitals (ruling 91/97) ;
- a Community decree requiring health-care institutions to develop an integral quality control system affects the accreditation of institutions, and thus falls within the jurisdiction of Communities. The court also held, however, that the decree did not limit the federal power to adopt norms of accreditation or basic norms governing hospitals. Consequently, both orders of government can proceed with some aspects of quality control in hospitals. However, the court noted that expenses arising from a Community decree must not burden the federal authorities.

This suggests that the constitutional court has intervened extensively in the field of health care. However, given that devolution occurred relatively recently in this highly developed area of public policy, the need for clarification is quite normal. Despite the detailed manner in which the distribution of powers was designed, it was impossible to anticipate every type of legislative and regulatory action. The process of clarification occurs on a regular basis at the political level, but the Court of Arbitration has thus been called upon to clarify grey areas. Partial devolution of an important sector of the welfare state requires a lot of fine-tuning, and both the judicial and political processes are involved in the exercise.

Intergovernmental Tensions in Health Care

Despite the mechanisms for cooperation and clarification, coordination between the federal government and the Communities has not been particularly easy and has represented a distinct challenge in two areas: health care for the elderly and education.

Since 1980, the Communities have enjoyed jurisdiction over public policy concerning "rest homes" for the elderly. They pass the framework legislation that sets planning and accreditation norms, and they have the obligation to subsidize the construction of such homes, which provide lodging and housekeeping care to persons over the age of 60. However, other public authorities have closely related powers. The federal Ministry of Economic Affairs must approve the charges to residents. Moreover, with the aging of the population, health care is increasingly important in these institutions. The federal health-care insurance plan grants a daily lump sum to cover health care provided by nursing staff and to help with daily activities and rehabilitation. To qualify for this financial contribution, the rest home must demonstrate that it has sufficient staff, based on the number of residents at every level of dependency.

The closing and conversion of hospital beds in the 1980s resulted in the creation of similar kinds of institutions: "rest and nursing homes." These institutions provide more health care than the simple rest homes, and are intended for persons who are affected by a long-lasting illness, but do not require daily medical regimes or specialized medical treatment. While rest homes come under Community jurisdiction, "rest and nursing homes" are governed by federal legislation, as is the case for hospitals. As a result, the basic regulation and operating costs are federal. As in the case of rest homes, the federal health-care insurance plan provides lump sums for nursing care and assistance with daily activities, and the federal Ministry of Economic Affairs approves accommodation costs. However, the Communities are responsible for infrastructure investment, accreditation, and programming within the federal framework. There is thus a very closely interwoven involvement of both orders of government in the running of those important institutions.

Another public policy initiative that is the subject of substantial debate in Belgium concerns the creation of a separate insurance plan for dependent elderly people, which some other European countries have already established. The new insurance scheme would cover non-medical costs facing dependent elderly people, such as housekeeping assistance and special equipment. According to some analysts, this new insurance would be an addition to the present social security system, and as such would fall under federal jurisdiction. For others, such "autonomy" insurance is "assistance to persons," which clearly comes under Community jurisdiction. Indeed, in the spring of 1999, the Flemish Parliament approved a decree introducing such insurance for the Flemish Community. The July 1999 program adopted by the new federal coalition government provides that there will be coordination between the federal level and the Communities, thus recognizing that both orders must play a role in this new social program.

Another area that requires coordination is medical education and access to the medical profession. While the Communities have had jurisdiction over the former since 1988, the federal government still has jurisdiction over the latter. In this context, it is the federal Ministry of Social Affairs and Health that determines the numbers of medical graduates admitted for specialization. As part of the effort to control health costs, a 1996 federal law introduced a *numerus clausus* for physicians and pharmacists to limit the number of new professionals. The federal government established the planning commission for medical supply discussed earlier, with representation of physicians, sickness funds, universities, the Communities, the federal ministry, and the NSIII. The commission agrees on quotas, which are divided between the Communities and then fixed by federal decree. A 1997 decree stipulates that the maximum number of physicians who will be able to obtain a professional qualification in 2004 will be 700, with 420 in the Flemish Community and 280 in the French-speaking Community.

While the quotas are set by federal regulation, the means of attaining these quotas are left to the Communities as part of their jurisdiction over education. The two Communities have chosen different paths: the Flemish Community has decided to organize a university entrance examination for medical studies, whereas the French-speaking Community has chosen to filter students in the course of their medical training, and to establish bridges to other studies for those who are excluded. This area is a good example of the interwoven nature of public action. The objective is negotiated by different orders of government and the relevant social partners, legislated by the federal government and implemented by the Communities.

This interwoven texture of jurisdiction not only creates a need for close coordination, it also makes the system as a whole sensitive to dynamism at any level. Although the overall power of the Communities is limited, the activism of the Flemish Community has had an important impact on federal programs and services. The Community has taken a number of initiatives concerning palliative care and screening for breast cancer, obliging the federal level to become more active in this domain. Another example concerns quality-control measures in hospitals. The Flemish Community introduced its own set of quality measures in parallel to federal norms. As mentioned earlier, the Court of Arbitration ruled that these two systems could constitutionally coexist, as long as the Community norms do not contradict federal ones and there is no impact on financing by the health insurance scheme. As a result, hospitals had to transfer a lot of information about their operations to the Community, which linked its contributions to capital investment to broadly-defined quality controls. Although the Flemish action technically focused on areas that were not being controlled by the federal authorities, it was also a way of getting involved in the management of hospitals and expanding the reality of Community power in health matters.

RECENT POLITICAL CONTROVERSIES

The current balance, in which some powers have been devolved to the Communities and health care remaining under federal jurisdiction, is increasingly seen as being unsatisfactory in Flemish circles. The result has been a continuing political tension that permeates a wide range of issues in health care, particularly on the role of interregional transfers, changes in the social security system, and constitutional reform.

Interregional Transfers

The role of interregional transfers has often been used as a lever in the Belgian discussion about the "defederalization" of health care; that is, the devolution of health care from the federal level to the Communities. Many opponents of the present centralized system deplore the financial transfers from Flanders to Wallonia that are implicit in social security in general, and the field of health care in particular. These transfers have been the object of charged political exchanges, and studies have repeatedly sought to assess the size of the transfers and the explanation for them.

The most important part of the financial transfer results from differences in salary and income levels between the two parts of the country. Incomes are higher in Flanders; and because social security contributions are proportional to salaries, they are also higher on a per capita basis in that region. North-south financial transfers are also partly explained by the difference in employment levels; since contributions are based on earnings, there are fewer contributors proportionately in Wallonia where unemployment is higher.

However, the source of interregional differences is not limited to financing, as per capita medical expenditure is also higher in the French part of the country. Regional differences in medical costs are not exclusively a Belgian phenomenon; they have been observed in many other countries. In the Begian debates, there is a broad consensus that transfers between different parts of the country, and the ensuing social solidarity that is sustained, are justified if they are based on "objective" factors, such as demographic differences (an older population, or one with a higher rate of fertility) or differences in rates of pathology (more occupational illness in Wallonia due to its industrial and mining past).

More controversy surrounds factors characterized as "subjective." They are arguably related to cultural preferences, and allegedly include more expensive medical practice in the French part of the country that results from differences in medical training, supply, and philosophy. Critics argue that francophones go more readily to specialists, and that French-speaking doctors order more medical tests than their Flemish counterparts. Many in Flanders insist that the Flemish population should not have to subsidize such cultural "preferences," which are not actually based on greater medical needs.

Both sides of the country recognized the need to examine the evidence more closely. First, the Flemish government commissioned a research team to examine "the transparency of financial transfers concerning social security and underlying mechanisms" in order to reduce transfers between Communities and Regions that cannot be explained on the basis of objective factors and therefore cannot be justified in the name of social solidarity. This research team wrote a detailed report with an important number of propositions, many of which have now been integrated into official Flemish Community political platforms.[13]

At the federal level, the General Council of the NSIII, the most important management body of the sickness insurance scheme, was entrusted in 1993 with writing an annual report on differences in the consumption of medical care, and proposing ways to eliminate differences that were not objective. To date, four reports have been transmitted to the federal government and examined by the federal parliament. The last report (January 2000), concluded that differences in medical consumption could not be explained fully by the social and health characteristics of the populations in different regions, and that there are regional differences in medical practices for a number of medical procedures. The report therefore calls for developing peer-review mechanisms and enhancing existing databases.

However, the reports also demonstrated that the political arguments about interregional differences were often simplistic and overstated. Table 3 sets out the ratio of average medical expenses by region, with the average for Belgium as a whole equal to 100.

These figures indicate that the highest average expenses occur in Brussels, which has an older population and greater medical supply than the rest of the country. In comparison, the differences between Flanders and Wallonia are more limited. Moreover, the analysis shows that certain differences within

TABLE 3
Ratio of Average Medical Expenditures (by region), 1997

	Flanders	*Wallonia*	*Brussels*
Ambulatory care	98	101	107
Hospital care	94	104	122
Total	96	102	115

Source: Data supplied by the National Sickness and Invalidity Insurance Institute, Brussels.

Regions, such as between rural and urban areas, are more important than differences between the Regions. The reports therefore constitute a partial response to the simplistic assertion that north-south transfers are caused by cultural differences, and that Flanders is being asked to subsidize expensive medical preferences in Wallonia.[14]

Calls for Reform of Social Security

A number of voices are calling for reform of the present social security system, in which entitlement to social benefits is largely based on the insured person's status in the labour market. Critics argue that some parts of the social security system, such as health care and family allowances, compensate citizens for basic needs and social obligations; as such, they should be available directly to the whole population, and should not be linked to one's employment status. The proposed reform would therefore establish two pillars within social security. The first pillar would provide cost-compensation programs such as health care and family allowance to the entire population. This pillar would be financed either through general taxation or earmarked contributions payable by the entire population. The second pillar would concern income-replacement programs, such as unemployment insurance and pensions. They would remain linked to employment and would continue to be financed by contributions proportional to salary.

Members of the Flemish Community have led the campaign for this proposal. It has not been implemented, however, for reasons unrelated to the basic logic of the policy ideas. The essential difficulty is that the issue triggers the debate about defederalization. Many argue that a "pillarization" of social security, and the separation of family allowances and health care from other branches of the system, would pave the way for the transfer of constitutional jurisdiction over those programs to the Communities. For example, the Flemish research group mentioned above suggested such a transfer and emphasized that, in order not to disrupt the Belgian economic union, devolution required the elimination of the link between the programs and employment status.[15] Many francophone politicians have opposed the reform proposals, not because they disagree with the basic policy ideas, but because of their constitutional consequences. In addition, the "social partners," who are intermediaries in the current social security system, oppose the reform for fear of losing influence in the process.

Constitutional Reforms

In 1996, the Flemish Parliament began to prepare the next stage of constitutional reform, the last one having occurred in 1993. The starting point was a discussion paper approved by the Flemish government on 29 February 1996, which included demands for a redistribution of powers in the health-care sector in order to create more homogeneous categories. In particular, the following areas were addressed:

- The need for increased coherence between preventive and healing care. It is argued that the potential financial advantages of an effective prevention policy must benefit the level of government that introduces and finances it; otherwise there is little incentive to implement effective preventative measures.
- The need for a better integration of medical care on the one hand and of welfare and elderly policy on the other.
- The need for Community modulation in health-care policy. The Flemish government holds that health care has a cultural dimension, and that regional differences in preferences concerning the organization of health care need to be accommodated. Recently, this has been summarized as: "the south chooses medicine, the north health care," a reference to the greater emphasis on specialized care in Wallonia and primary care in Flanders.

The debate concerning the 1996 discussion paper lasted three years and led to the adoption of a certain number of resolutions by the Flemish Parliament on 3 March 1999. The implementation of a more coherent constitutional distribution of powers is considered a priority objective for the next stage of constitutional reform. Concerning health care, the Flemish resolutions held that:

> the legislative power, as well as powers of implementation and financing of the whole of health-care policy must be completely transferred to the federated entities, including the health-care insurance plan (which is a cost-compensation program). The inhabitants of the Region of Brussels-Capital must be free to choose between the Flemish system and the system for the French-speakers, which would be distinct from the point of view of financing, as well as expenditure. [Our translation]

The response of the federal government has been much more cautious. An assessment of the new federal structures was launched as a result of the June 1995 agreement of the incoming coalition government. The government recognized that the new federal structures were "dynamic" and that an examination of possible improvements to the distribution of powers, institutions, or means of cooperation would be useful. The Senate was charged with this assessment, which began in 1996. A detailed report was released on 30 March 1999, setting forth an inventory of suggestions. In the case of health care, the report gives very little detail, and mostly pleads for the development of more functional cooperation between orders of government.

The fundamental reason for the slow pace is powerful resistance from Wallonia. Proposals to "communitarize" health care have received a negative response from the French-speaking population and political leaders, who fear that splitting jurisdiction would lead to a weakening of social solidarity. As it is currently organized, Belgian social security rests on a form of solidarity between persons, not between Regions or Communities. They insist that the existing differences in health expenditures are not culturally or linguistically linked, but are primarily driven by objective differences in income generated by economic forces such as the major economic crisis in Wallonia and the growth of poverty in Brussels, or by differences in the health status that are a legacy of the history of heavy industry in the south. Finally, many Walloon representatives insist that splitting, even partially, the present social security system could actually trigger the end of Belgium as a united country, because of the polarization it would induce in a very sensitive domain of public life.

This conflict was not resolved, as many Flemish advocates had hoped, by the outcome of the 1999 federal election. The issue of reorganization of health care was not directly addressed in the process of forming the federal coalition government in July of that year. The coalition partners simply "agreed to agree" on a procedure for further discussions about reforms to state structures.

In the end, the government established an intergovernmental and inter-parliamentary conference, with linguistic parity in its membership and two presidents, one Dutch-speaking and one French-speaking. The conference included representatives of the governments and parliaments of the federal, Community, and Regional levels. However, consensus on health care remained illusive. The conference deferred tackling the issue, and the formal process of constitutional reform finally triggered in 1991 did not include health care.

THE FUTURE OF FEDERALISM AND HEALTH CARE IN BELGIUM

Belgian health policy remains at a crossroads. Although the subject has been deferred again, it has not gone away. The challenge remains to find a balance between subsidiarity, efficient administration and transparent solidarity. Until now, discussion of the *communautarisation* of health care has mainly been carried out in academic circles and among political parties. Several important social partners in the field have not taken a clear position, fearing that bold and radical changes might challenge their position in the system. In the meantime, some policy reforms have been blocked, in part because of fears of the consequences on the constitutional front. As we have seen, the growing body of opinion that family allowances and health care should be disassociated from the professional status of the person and granted to the whole population is resisted by those who fear that the reform project is really a forerunner of the transfer of health care to the Communities and the erosion of social solidarity in Belgium. The evolution of health care in many countries has involved a trend toward decentralization, and it remains unclear whether Belgium will escape this evolution. All that can be asserted with confidence at this stage is that the issue of federalism and health care will continue to feature prominently in debates over Belgium's future.

NOTES

[1]In the context of a country that becomes federal by decentralization of a unitary state, opposed to the reunion of distinct entities in one polity, "federalization" means "to make federal" or "to decentralize." In Belgium the expression is used interchangeably with *communautarisation* (a transfer to Communities) or "regionalization" (a transfer to Regions).

[2]Regional decrees of the Walloon parliament also apply in the German-speaking area. However, in the case of community matters, the German-speaking community has its own parliament, which has 25 seats.

[3]Which, with some nuances, have the same authority as federal law or "decrees" adopted by the other federated entities.

[4]For instance, the minister-president of the Walloon Region was, until the spring of 2000, also president of the federal French-speaking Socialist Party, which is a member of the federal coalition government.

[5]However, the representatives of the federal government do retain a veto power on financial decisions.

[6]Article 6, section 1 of the 1980 *Special Institutional Reform Act*, as amended in 1988.

[7]A number of these officials were working in the Department of Public Health on environmental matters which became a regional competence at the same time.

[8]See article 5, section 1 of the same Act.

[9]Since 1994, the Walloon Region, the French-speaking Region, and the French Community Commission (COCOF), and the bilingual Region of the Brussels-Capital, have exercised the authority of the French Community over health-care policy, except for academic hospitals, the Centre hospitalier de l'Université de Liège, the Belgian Royal academy of Medicine, the Office national de l'enfance (ONE), sanitary education, activities and services of preventive medicine and for medical inspection in schools. The competences fall under the jurisdiction of the Communities.

[10]Again, in the French area of the country, the exercise of powers was regionalized in 1994.

[11]The Council of State, a federally-appointed administrative court, has two sections. The "legislation section" reviews all federal, Community, and Regional legislative measures before their adoption to ensure, amongst other things, that they respect the distribution of powers. The "administrative section" can rule on the constitutionality of regulations after they have been adopted (in the case of legislation, this role is played by the Court of Arbitration). While the Council of State is a federal institution, each section is subdivided into two linguistic chambers which function independently from one another.

[12]This is a kind of reference jurisdiction, but in favour of courts, rather than the executive as is the case in Canada.

[13]D. Pieters, ed., *Juridisch onderzoek naar de financiële transfers in de sociale zekerheid,* deel 1, Vlaamse Onderzoeksgroep, Sociale Zekerheid, Leuven 1994.

[14]In the scope of a new system that renders sickness funds *partly* responsible financially, a research team appointed by the federal government has been entrusted with explaining the interregional differences in medical expenses, according to individual health-care data. This research is still ongoing. Its results should help the NSIII distribute financial means between the sickness funds according to specified objective risk factors, as opposed to total actual expenses, as is the case today.

[15]Otherwise, employers in the north and south might have to pay different contributions for those programs, which could introduce economic disruption and delocalization.

3

FEDERALISM AND THE GERMAN HEALTH-CARE SYSTEM

Dietmar Wassener

INTRODUCTION

The German constitution defines Germany as "a democratic and social federal state." Both federalism and a system of social security are therefore constituent elements of German society, and the German social-security system including health care is organized to some extent according to federal principles. Federalism, however, is often superseded by other fundamental principles of the German social-security system. Recent reforms, such as the *Structural Health Reform Act*, have kindled a debate on the necessity of more federalism within the social-security system and more regionalism within the German health-care system. However, this chapter will show that, while the health-care system will undoubtedly undergo further structural reforms, the basic ideas that define the German health-care system — self-administration, subsidiarity, and solidarity — are unlikely to be questioned or altered. In comparison, federalism will continue to play a secondary role in shaping German health care.

The German Federal System: Interlocking Federalism

Germany as a federal state consists of 16 states or *Länder*, each with its own government and parliament. On the national level, the federal government or Bundesregierung acts as the executive body. The federal parliament has two chambers: the Bundestag or lower house whose members are elected directly in nationwide elections; and the Bundesrat, the upper house which consists of representatives from the 16 state governments.[1]

One of the main features of the German federation is a system of *interlocking federalism* which results from several factors: the constitutional distribution of powers, a highly integrated fiscal system, and the role that the Bundesrat plays in federal legislation. In theory, article 30 of the German constitution provides significant legislative powers for the states. In practice, however, "the wide array of concurrent legislation has to all intents and purposes been absorbed by the federal level of government, with the consequence of limiting the legislative powers of the Länder to a small number of exclusive powers."[2] This dominance of the federal government in the field of concurrent powers is especially true in the field of social policy where the states have very little exclusive legislative competence. Nevertheless, the states are directly involved in much of the legislative policy-making on the federal level through their role in the Bundesrat. Indeed, the very term "federal" in Germany always includes not only the Bundesregierung and the Bundestag but also the states as represented in the Bundesrat.

The mechanism of interlocking federalism ensures that the states are involved in all aspects of policy implementation. All federal laws have to be considered by the *Bundesrat* and many need its approval. For example, article 77 of the constitution requires approval for those laws that affect the interests of the states such as financial matters or administration. Today, more than 60 percent of all federal laws have to be approved by the upper house of parliament. The Bundesrat plays an important part in coordinating both orders of government. Through this independent institution, states do not only participate in the federal legislation but also in the administrative procedures of the federal government. In cases of conflict between Bundestag and the Bundesrat over legislation needing the Bundesrat's approval, a mediation committee (*Vermittlungsauschuß*) consisting of members of both parliamentary chambers is installed to resolve the disputes.

The system of interlocking federalism is also reflected in the tax system. While legislative sovereignty for determining taxes lies predominantly with the federal government, the tax revenues are distributed among the federal, state, and local levels according to independent principles operating through complicated mechanisms. These mechanisms include vertical transfers between the federal level and the states, horizontal transfers among states themselves, and local transfers among communities.[3] In 1997, about DM12 billion were transferred between states through the horizontal interstate tax transfer system alone, with DM 5.3 billion going to the east German states.[4] While the present system is criticized by some states, this criticism explicitly does not include the interregional solidarity with the east German states whose need for further financial support is generally acknowledged. Nevertheless, the effects of the fiscal crisis brought on by the costs of unification are putting this system of intergovernmental relations under some strain, as it tends to reduce the flexibility of both orders of government and therefore reduces, rather than increases, the speed of necessary reforms.[5]

The tax-transfer mechanisms are laid out in the constitution. Compared to other federal systems, the freedom of both the federal and state governments to raise revenues independently is small. The formal competence of the state governments in the area of tax legislation are extremely small; and the freedom of the federal government to raise revenues independently is restricted because it depends on the consent of the majority in the Bundesrat to changes in any tax law that directly affects the state revenues.

The interlocking nature of German federalism gives the system a strongly corporatist dimension which is reflected in a number of intergovernmental consensus mechanisms. Coordination between the different orders of government takes place in all the various stages of the process of policy development and implementation. There are formal and informal meetings vertically between representatives of the federal and state governments, and on the horizontal level among representatives of the states without the involvement of the federal government.[6] Furthermore, there are hundreds of working parties on all political levels, ranging from the heads of government and departmental ministers to the departmental officers at the sectoral level.

The complexity of the interlocking German federalism and its corporate structures directly influence decision-making. The system in most cases leads to a relatively high degree of political consensus and stability between the various levels of government. But the complex consensus mechanisms also tend to obstruct policy initiatives aimed at solving the complicated problems that are most likely to be found in the welfare system.[7] This is especially true in the case of a "divided government," when different political parties control the two houses of parliament. In such periods, decisions can only be taken with the backing of a majority of conservatives and social-democrats. This kind of political stalemate existed between 1994 and 1998, with a liberal-conservative majority in the Bundestag, and a social-democrat majority in the Bundesrat. After a brief interlude following the 1998 election when the Social Democrats controlled both houses, divided government returned in 1999 when they lost control of the Bundesrat. The result has been that the German federal government was free to lead only in the field of foreign and defence policy, whereas domestic and especially social policy has become a domain of the *Vermittlungsauchuss* between both chambers of parliament.

In this system, it is hard to define precisely the ultimate source of leadership. However, fundamental political decisions of national importance — such as a general restructuring of the statutory health insurance — are taken at the national level. In most cases, the federal government initiates the legislative process, usually in consensus with state governments led by the same political party in order to ensure some support in the Bundesrat. Its proposals are then discussed and often modified in both chambers of parliament. Defining precisely the source of political leadership is even harder in the field of social policy.[8] In the social-security system, the cooperation and coordination implicit in interlocking federalism are supplemented by corporatist relationships with representatives of employers and employees. These relationships are organized according to fundamental principles of their own, including subsidiarity, solidarity, and self-administration by the "social partners," with important consequences for the decision-taking process.

Principles of the German Social-Security System

Although the German social-security system is in many aspects organized along federal lines, federalism is not its basic principle. Questions of federalism tend to be superseded by the discussion about the shape of solidarity and the level at which a uniformity of living conditions should be achieved and maintained.

The German welfare system dates back to the second half of the nineteenth century.[9] The first health-insurance law was adopted in 1883, the basis for occupational accident insurance was laid in 1884, a statutory pension insurance was founded in 1889, unemployment insurance was introduced in 1927, and a fifth branch of the insurance system — nursing insurance — was finally added in 1994. The basic principles of the German social insurance system are:[10]

- The *insurance principle*. By paying contributions to the insurance system insured individuals earn claims on benefits. These benefits may be based on individual needs, as in the case of health insurance, or on individual financial contributions, for example, pension and unemployment insurance.

- The *principle of self-administration within a legal framework.* The self-administration of the social funds for health insurance, pensions, and so on is a central principle of the German social system. While the federal government sets the legal framework through the Social Code, it is employers and employees who actually administer the different social insurance plans through representatives' assemblies and executive boards in which both employees and employers are equally represented. In the case of the health sector, these legally independent, demand-side organizations face equally independent, self-administered, supply-side organizations of physicians and hospitals.
- The *principle of organizational diversity* within the branches of social security. While organizational diversity is largely a result of historical development, it is widely accepted today. In the health sector, for example, this principle would never allow a single, nationwide insurance plan. Instead, it leads to a highly decentralized structure of statutory health-care funds.

These insurance principles are complemented by the *principle of public assistance.* The state intervenes in those cases where insurance turns out to be insufficient because no contributions are being paid or because the legal framework does not provide coverage through insurance.

Under these principles, social security in Germany is provided to a large extent by statutory insurance financed through contributions rather than by the state through taxes.[11] In those fields where social security is provided by the insurance system, the role of government — both federal or regional — is limited to setting the legal framework. Discussions about federalism and regionalism within the German social-security system are therefore often transferred from the governmental sector (federal government versus state governments) to the insurance sector (nationwide versus regional calculation of contribution rates, nationwide or regional organizational structures).

In order to understand the German social-security system and the current debate on regionalism within this system, it is important to examine the role of subsidiarity and solidarity as they are understood in Germany. The social-security system reflects the principle of *subsidiarity*, which holds that social functions such as health care should, whenever possible, be taken care of by the smallest social unit and should be delegated upwards to larger units only if the smaller unit proves unable to fulfil the function. Although the family is regarded as the nucleus of society, when it proves unable to cover risks such as illness, it is the solidarity within the association of the insured that provides the necessary coverage. In this view, the state should intervene only when the insurance system fails to provide security. It is also argued that whatever social aspects can be regulated on a state level should not be delegated to the federal level.

Subsidiarity is complemented by *solidarity*. In the German view, solidarity means that costs and benefits should be broadly shared among all the groups and members of society. While solidarity within the social-security system primarily refers to the solidarity among members of a single insurance fund, the concept of solidarity also applies nationwide and is, for example, reflected in the significant financial transfers from west to east Germany within the unemployment insurance system and the pension plan.[12] In the health-care sector, the idea of solidarity is most clearly seen within each statutory health-insurance fund. The fund's contribution rate is calculated as a percentage of wages, leading to higher absolute contributions by wealthier persons, while benefits are provided strictly according to need. While this element of solidarity occurs within individual funds, other elements of the system also reflect the principle of solidarity on a wider basis. Health policy changes are widely negotiated, and consensus is sought between all concerned parties including the providers, individual funds, and policymakers. Financial transfers between funds are also common. The risk-equalization mechanism, which is discussed in greater detail below, leads to significant transfers between funds and adds an element of inter-fund solidarity. Finally, solidarity also depends on a complex series of rights and obligations involving providers, insurers, governments, and other parties. These rights and obligations are clearly reflected in the German health-insurance law, in the delegation of responsibility for the system's administration to physician associations, sickness funds, and other groups. In effect, solidarity is "the basis on which the structure is built, and which binds it together."[13]

The German Health Care System

The framework of the German health-care system is depicted in Figure 1, which provides a simplified view of the flows of finances and health benefits within the system. As noted earlier, any discussion on federalism and regionalism concentrates less on intergovernmental relations and more on the relationships and organizational structures of the self-governing provider associations and health-insurance funds. In this respect, the main participants in the German

FIGURE 1
Main Transactions within the German Health-Care System

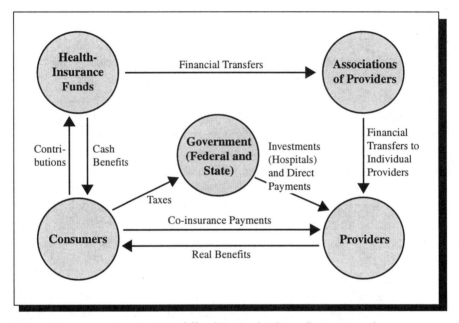

Source: Presentation based on M. Pfaff and F. Nagel, "Gesundheitssysteme der Europäischen Gemeinschaft im Vergleich," *Das Gesundheitswesen* 56, 2 (1994):86-91.

health-care system are the federal and state governments, the provider associations (including ambulatory care physicians and hospitals), and the health-insurance funds.

Given the traditions of the German welfare state, the organization and financing of health care are to a large extent transferred from the government to the self-administering health-insurance funds and provider associations. The calculation of contribution rates, the setting of prices for health services, and the definition of benefits paid for by the insurance funds and therefore provided by doctors are all left mostly to self-administration. The role of the federal and state governments is reduced largely to setting the legal framework for the interaction between the partners of the self-administration system. This includes, for example, defining the principles of how to calculate contribution rates, setting minimal standards for benefits to be provided, or — possibly the most drastic "intrusion" into the system of self-administration — defining an overall maximum budget for health expenditures.

The legal framework is set, with few exceptions, on the federal level through the regulations of the Social Code.[14] The constitutional distribution of powers within the German health-care sector provides that both the federal and state governments, or their legislative bodies, are engaged in the task of setting health-policy goals, formulating general guidelines, and controlling adherence to the legal framework. The Federal Insurance Bureau supervises those health-insurance funds organized on a federal level such as the substitute funds, the miners' fund, and the private health-insurance plans. The federal Health Ministry is responsible for the federal organizations of the health-insurance funds and also controls a number of health authorities such as the Federal Bureau for Food Control and Federal Centre for Health Education. The state governments are responsible for the Public Health Offices, which provide for health promotion and disease control and supervise the regional and local health-insurance funds. Furthermore, and most importantly, hospital planning is the responsibility of the state governments, which finance investments in the hospital sector from their tax revenues.

Ambulatory-care physicians are organized into associations. Physicians receive their remuneration from their own associations, which submit the claims of individual doctors to the health-insurance funds. There are general contracts at the federal and state levels for the delivery and monitoring of medical services, and for providing the general framework for the relationship between the health-insurance funds and the health-insurance-fund physicians. These general contracts regulate the particulars of the medical services rendered, principles of reimbursements, fees for services, processing of claims, and economic monitoring.

Although the general guidelines are mostly outlined at a federal level, reimbursement is calculated at the state level. The state associations of ambulatory-care physicians control both the right of physicians to practise in the region, and the reimbursement of fees that are negotiated with the state associations of health-insurance funds. Each ambulatory-care physician submits vouchers for patients of the sickness funds to the regional association for reimbursement. The association itself monitors the volume and value of services of each physician and controls the number and value of prescriptions and referrals.[15]

Hospitals are organized rather loosely. The state hospital associations and the German Hospital Association represent the interests of individual institutions. Since these institutions hold the status of private associations, however, they cannot regulate the conduct of an individual hospital. Moreover, since public, private non-profit, and private for-profit hospitals coexist, their interests differ considerably, which constrains effective organization of the sector. The German hospital sector is financed in a dual fashion: investment is funded by the state government, while the variable costs are covered by the health-insurance funds. As a result, conflicts can arise over the responsibility for financing investment in buildings and equipment. Furthermore, although hospital planning is the responsibility of the state governments, the health-insurance funds can terminate their contracts with particular hospitals if problems in quality arise or if an economically sound hospital operation is not maintained.

All in all, the distribution of power between state governments and health-insurance funds is rather delicate in this sector. Although conflicts between state governments and health-insurance funds arise mostly at the regional or state level, they can develop an interregional dimension in cases where access to hospital services is not restricted to a single state. For example, although the services of the Hamburg hospitals are also available to patients from the states of Niedersachsen and Schleswig-Holstein, only the citizens of the state of Hamburg contribute to investment in buildings and equipment through their taxes.[16]

One possible solution to this conflict between financial and planning interests would be a "monistic" financing structure. Under this model, the health-insurance funds would finance both investment and the running costs of the hospital sector, and in return would be solely responsible for hospital planning. While neither the *Structural Health Reform Act* of 1993 nor the recent *Restructuring Acts* of 1997 included legislative steps in this direction, the current draft by Social Democrats and Greens for a reform of the statutory health insurance (*GKV-Gesundheitsreform 2000*) proposes the introduction of a monistic financing system in three steps by the year 2008.

German federal legislation requires that employees have health insurance, regardless of their income. In 1995 about 9 percent of the population was insured by private health-insurance plans, while nearly 90 percent of the population was insured in the statutory health-insurance system.[17] In the statutory system, contributions are calculated as a percentage of gross wages up to a nationally defined-income ceiling, which determines the maximum contribution. The contribution rate for statutory health insurance averaged about 13.5 percent in 1998 (see Figure 5 below) and is shared equally between employer and employee.

A large number of insurance funds provide the statutory health-insurance package. In 1995, these included 17 general funds (AOK), 677 company-based funds, 93 guild- or craft-based funds, 19 agricultural funds, one seamen's and one miners' fund, and 15 so-called substitute health-insurance plans.[18] About 90 percent of the total population are insured by these more than 800 health-insurance funds. All employees under a defined-income limit, unemployed persons, pensioners, self-employed farmers, disabled persons, students, and artists are covered by statutory health-insurance funds.

The organizational structure of the statutory health-insurance funds is mostly decentralized and varies widely (see Figure 2).[19] About 45 percent of all members of the statutory insurance system are insured through insurance plans on the federal level, while the rest are insured through funds organized on a local or regional level.[20]

The general or local funds (AOK) were, until recently, organized on a regional level, leading to about 270 general funds in west Germany alone. They calculated their contribution rates on this regional basis, with the result that persons insured with a general fund in Munich might pay a different contribution rate than somebody living and working in Hamburg. Following the *Structural Reform Act* of 1993, most general insurance funds underwent a restructuring process which led to organizations at the state level and a statewide calculation of contribution rates. In 1995, about 42 percent of all members of statutory insurance plans were insured in these general funds.

Company-based insurance funds are mostly organized strictly on a company level, and traditionally only company employees and their families are insured in these funds. This principle leads to a local organizational structure, but the funds of larger companies operating nationwide often calculate their contribution rates on a national level. These represent about 17 percent of all company-based funds and cover about 42 percent of members of company-based plans. Following the *Structural Reform Act* of 1993, company-based insurance funds are no longer restricted to company employees, but may include non-company members. This is also true of guild-based funds, which can choose to no longer restrict themselves to the craft sector. The market share of company-based insurance funds is about 11 percent. Guild-based funds, which have about 6 percent of the market, are basically the health-insurance funds of craftspersons. They used to be organized on a local level but, as a result of the *Structural Reform Act* of 1993, most guild-based funds have now fused at the state level.

Finally, the substitute funds, which until 1995 were restricted mostly to white-collar workers, are organized on a federal level, differentiating only between west and east Germany — a result of the prevailing differences in incomes of employees. Their contribution rates are calculated at the federal

FIGURE 2
Organizational Structures of the German Statutory Health-Insurance Funds

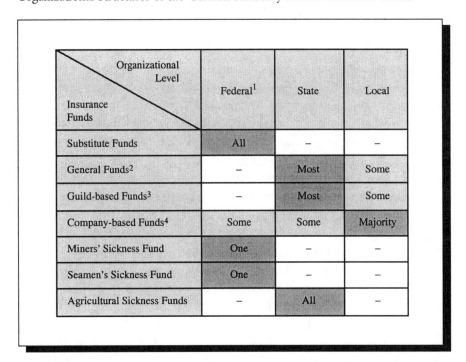

Insurance Funds \ Organizational Level	Federal[1]	State	Local
Substitute Funds	All	–	–
General Funds[2]	–	Most	Some
Guild-based Funds[3]	–	Most	Some
Company-based Funds[4]	Some	Some	Majority
Miners' Sickness Fund	One	–	–
Seamen's Sickness Fund	One	–	–
Agricultural Sickness Funds	–	All	–

Notes: [1]All health-insurance funds differentiate between east and west Germany.
[2]General funds in North-Rhine-Westphalia and Saxony-Anhalt are not organized at a strictly state level.
[3]Guild-based funds used to be organized at a local level mostly. Now most funds are organized at a state level.
[4]The company sickness funds of larger companies often calculate their contribution rates on a federal or state level. Accordingly about 17 percent of all company sickness funds (with about 42 percent of the insured members) are not organized at a local level.

Source: Author's compilation.

level. About 36 percent of all members of statutory insurance plans are insured in substitute funds.

All statutory health-insurance funds are committed to basic principles laid out in the Social Code. The principle of solidarity (*Solidarprinzip*) specifies that medical attention should be provided purely on the basis of individual needs, whereas financing should be paid for according to the individual's financial ability. This principle leads to redistributive effects not only between the healthy and the sick, but also between single individuals and families (family members are insured without having to pay premiums), employees earning high wages and those earning little (the contribution rate is calculated as a percentage of gross wages), and between the young and the old (the latter on average being sick more often).

Historically, the principle of solidarity limited redistribution within statutory health insurance to these dimensions. The principle did not foresee interregional redistribution, nor did it engage differences in financial burdens that emerge solely as a result of individuals being insured in different funds. The question arising here is whether solidarity within the statutory health-insurance fund should be defined on a nationwide level or whether each of the 800 health-insurance funds is the relevant basis for solidarity. A nationwide definition of solidarity implies a risk-equalization mechanism on a federal level, which is discussed below. Defining the 15 German states as the relevant general risk pools would lead to a strengthening of regional responsibilities and would require calculating all contribution rates on a regional or state level.[21]

The principle of economy in the SGB V (*Sozialgesetzbuch*) holds that both insurance funds and providers are responsible for economically sound structures and an adequate but not excessive supply of health services. The *Structural Reform Act* of 1993 stresses this principle of economy, as it includes measures to increase competition among health-insurance funds in order to increase efficiency and effectiveness. As competition among health-care providers, as well as among health-insurance funds has to take place on a regional level, the strengthening of competition implies a shifting of responsibilities away from the federal level on both the supply and the demand side.

The third principle is self-administration within the health sector. As pointed out above, the German welfare system is largely an insurance-based system. The statutory health-care insurance plans are self-administering. They are independent not only as to their organizational structure and the calculation of their contribution rates; in agreement with the health-care providers, they are also responsible to a large extent for deciding which health services are allotted. The principle of self-administration is seldom challenged directly because of the political power of the health-care administrations. The highly decentralized structure of the statutory health-care funds and the relatively small direct influence of both federal and state governments is largely a result of the principle of self-administration.

Within this system, there is no standardized mechanism for solving disputes. Rather, a complex system of cooperation has developed. For example, while funds may compete for the insured on a local level, they cooperate on the national level when negotiating remuneration with the physicians' associations. In addition, both the physicians' associations and the federal organizations representing the funds, although often bitter opponents in other matters, collectively define the catalogue of medical benefits considered useful and necessary and therefore paid for by the insurance plans. Disputes within the self-administration system are usually solved through negotiations or by arbitration committees consisting of members of both provider organizations and funds. Unresolvable disputes may be brought before the social affairs courts. Interestingly, German law does not provide for intervention of the federal Health Ministry in cases of disputes between providers and health-insurance agencies. The Social Code restricts governmental control to supervisory tasks such as accountancy and quality control.

On the government side, there are no special institutions for the resolution of federal versus state disputes in the health-care sector. For example, there is no official intergovernmental committee of health ministers. Disputes are resolved through general intergovernmental mechanisms such as the mediation committee that deals with conflicts between the two houses of parliament.

Finally, a permanent committee entitled Concerted Action for Health Care brings together all the actors in the health-care sector, including federal and state governments, to discuss potential disputes and necessary reforms. Its function is to mediate in cases of conflict and to discuss possibilities for health-care reform. The committee is supported by an advisory council of independent scientists, and it may make recommendations. However, this body has no legislative or executive powers.

Financing Health Care in Germany

The German health-care system is often described as a social insurance model characterized by an almost universal and compulsory coverage.[22] However, it is probably better defined as a "mixed system" that is financed through contributions from both by employees and employers, through co-insurance payments of the insured in case of illness, and through general taxes.

Contributions account for about 60 percent of financial resources. These resources are channelled by the associations of health-insurance funds to the associations of providers; and the latter distribute the funds to the individual providers in line with the latter's claims for the health services they have provided. The public sector (federal, state, and local governments) finances both the purely public health institutions such as the public health service, and the fixed costs of public hospitals such as investment in buildings and equipment. The variable hospital costs, related to services provided to the insured, are paid for by the health-insurance funds from the contributions paid by their members.[23]

Most of these contributions, calculated as a percentage of wages earned, are paid on a 50/50 basis by employers and employees. Various exceptions to this rule, such as occupational accident insurance and private health insurance, however, lead to higher contributions paid by private households (DM 181 billion) as compared to employers (DM 126 billion).

As shown in Figure 3, the statutory health-insurance system forms the backbone of the financing of the German health sector. In 1996, nearly half of the DM 525 billion transferred within the health sector were channelled through statutory health-insurance funds.[24] Excluding the direct cash transfers (mostly pensions and sick-pay[25]) highlights the importance of the statutory health-insurance system even further. Of the DM 388 billion transferred to insurance plans covering health costs in 1996, DM 244 billion (72 percent) went to statutory health-insurance funds, which insured about 90 percent of the population. Health expenditures were also covered by pension plans (DM 38 billion), private health insurance (DM 27 billion), and nursing and occupational accident insurance (DM 15 billion).

Compared to the statutory health-insurance system, the public sector plays a secondary role. All in all, governments contributed DM 103 billion tax-financed revenues to the health-care sector. This includes about DM 39 billion (mostly state-paid contributions for pensioners) that were transferred to the insurance plans to cover health costs. Only DM 64 billion (12 percent of total health expenditures) were delivered directly by the federal, state, and local governments. These included payments for the costs of rehabilitative measures (DM 18.8 billion), the payment of contributions for nursing insurance for the recipients of public assistance (DM 14.2 billion), medical education (DM 8.8 billion), and investment by state governments in the hospital sector (DM 13.7 billion).

Private households contribute to financing health care in two ways. In 1996, they paid contributions of about DM 181 billion to health-insurance plans,

FIGURE 3
Financing Health Care in Germany, Data for 1996

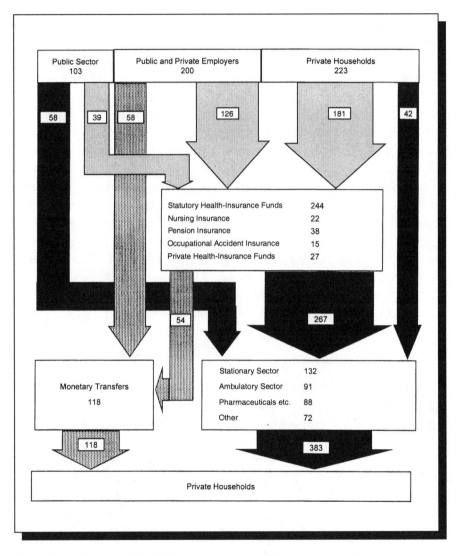

Note: Not depicted are DM 6 billion in monetary transfers from the public sector to the private households, DM 16 billion in direct transfers from the employers to the health sectors and DM 25 billion of administration costs of the health institutions (insurance).

Source: Author's compilation based on data from the German Statistical Office. See W. Müller, "Ausgaben für Gesundheit 1996," *Soziale Sicherheit* 47, 11 (1998):915-23.

and their co-payments (e.g., for pharmaceuticals and hospital treatments) and private expenditures (e.g. for pharmaceuticals not paid for by insurance) added up to about DM 42 billion.

With the unification of Germany in 1989, the west German health-care system was introduced in the new east German Länder. The health-care structures of the former German Democratic Republic, including polyclinics and civil-servant physicians, were completely dissolved. In order for the east German health-care structures to reach west German levels of availability, coverage, and quality huge investments were necessary. The restructuring of the ambulatory sector through the establishment of independent physicians' practices was financed primarily through commercial credit institutions. The necessary investment in the hospital sector was calculated to be somewhere between DM 26 billion and DM 34 billion.[26] This funding had to be provided by the east German states, who in turn received significant financial transfers through the horizontal tax-transfer system and the "German Unity Fund." Furthermore, west German statutory insurance funds loaned DM 1 billion to east German funds in 1997 alone in order to subsidize them. In 1999 DM 1.2 billion were transferred from west German funds to the east German statutory insurance via the new national equalization mechanism for income differences of members of the statutory health-insurance system.

RECENT TRENDS

As in most other industrialized states, the ever-increasing cost of health care in Germany are considered to be a major financial and social problem. Indeed, since the mid-1970s most health-care reforms have been stimulated by the need for cost containment, although recent reforms such as the *Structural Reform Act* of 1993 have also induced structural changes affecting both providers and consumers in the health-care sector. More importantly in the context of this chapter, these reforms have also affected the structure of statutory health-care insurance and caused significant intra- and interregional transfers between the German states through the risk-equalization mechanism.

Health-Care Costs and Contribution Rates

The German health-care system is considered to be highly effective in providing high-quality services to almost the entire population. For example, there is no evidence of official or unofficial waiting lists of any kind for hospital admission. Only 6 percent of Germans reported having to wait more than one week to see a doctor in 1994, as compared to 15 percent in the United States and 16 percent in Canada.[27] Nevertheless, the German health-care sector has been characterized by significant increases in costs for decades. Cost-containment efforts such as the *Health Reform Act* of 1989 failed to turn this trend around: as Figure 4 indicates, overall costs covered by the statutory insurance system in west Germany increased from about DM 160 billion in 1991 to DM 206 billion in 1998, and east Germany added about DM 42 billion.

Expenditures rose in all sectors of the health-care system. For example, in 1992, the year before the *Structural Reform Act* was enacted, costs for ambulatory physicians rose by 8 percent in west Germany. In the same year, hospital costs rose by 8.3 percent and expenditures for phamaceuticals increased by 9.1 percent. Overall health expenditures rose by 9.2 percent, and health expenditures in east Germany rose even more dramatically.[28]

FIGURE 4
Total Expenditures of the German Statutory Health Insurance

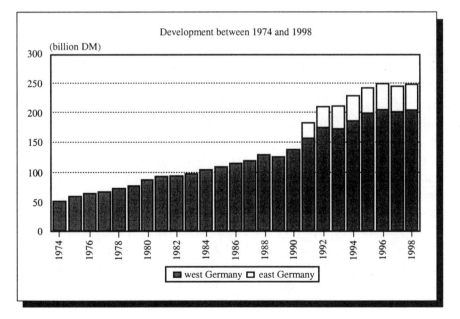

Source: Author's compilation based on data of the German Health Ministry (see: <www.bmgesundheit.de>).

Although these increases were substantial, they are by no means extraordinary. Neither the increases in health expenditures nor the ratio of health expenditures to the gross national product (GNP) exceeds international comparisons. In 1997, 10.4 percent of the German GNP was spent in the health sector. In the same year the numbers for other industrialized countries were: Canada 9.3 percent, France 9.9 percent, and the United States 14 percent.[29]

Increasing health expenditures were not the only reason — probably not even the main reason — for the Reform Act of 1993. Far more worrisome to politicians and experts alike were the constantly increasing contribution rates to the statutory health-insurance funds. These increases were caused by the discrepancy between the rate of increase in health expenditures and the rate of increase in gross wages, which determines the incomes accessible to the insurance funds as a basis for calculating contribution rates.[30] Over the last decade health expenditures have risen faster than gross wages. In 1992, for example, the incomes of members of statutory insurance funds rose by 7.7 percent, while expenditures increased by 9.2 percent. Since the contribution rates of the funds are calculated as a ratio between expenditures and the gross earnings of its members, this process automatically increases contribution rates. Morever, because the share of wages in GNP was declining, the financial base of health insurance — the wages of workers — was narrowing in this period. The resulting growth in contribution rates, highlighted in Figure 5, was, and still is, highly unpopular not only with policymakers and employees, but also with employers who pay half of the contributions to the health-insurance funds.

Because of the decentralized structure of most German statutory health-insurance funds, contribution rates vary widely: every one of the 800 insurance plans calculates its own contribution rate as a ratio between expenditures and the gross earnings of its members. Accordingly, rates are far from equal, as Figure 5 indicates. While the average contribution rate for all statutory health-insurance funds was 12.7 percent in 1992, contribution rates of individual funds varied between 16.5 percent (a general fund) and 8.5 percent (a company-based fund). Rates for general funds are, on average, higher than those for company-based or substitute funds. As a result, many Germans pay substantially more for health coverage, but receive essentially the same benefits as those who pay less. Moreover, these differences have been growing. Increases in average contribution rates parallel an ever-increasing range of contribution rates, which in turn signify increasing differences in the amount paid monthly for health coverage.

FIGURE 5
Contribution Rates in the German Statutory Health Insurance

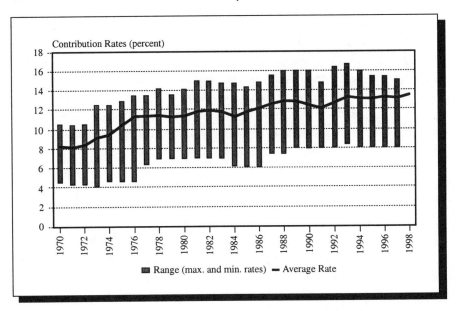

Source: Author's compilation based on data from the German Health Ministry.

Contribution rates also vary widely between states. While the 1995 contribution rate of the general fund in Baden-Württemberg was 12.9 percent, it was 15.5 percent in Hamburg.[31] For politicians, especially those from states with high average contribution rates, these differences were not in accordance with the fundamental principle of equal living conditions within the German federal system. They also conflicted with the principle of solidarity, which holds that the distributive effects of the financing mechanism should be limited to the individual's financial abilities and should not include differences resulting from being insured by different funds or by living in different states.[32]

To summarize, the major problems facing the German health-care system in the 1970s and 1980s were rising costs and increasing differences in contribution rates which violated the fundamental principle of solidarity and equal living conditions. Policymakers have reacted by concentrating on cost reduction and, in 1993, on structural reforms aimed at both increasing efficiency and restoring solidarity.

Policy Goals

Since the mid-1970s, health-care reforms have been mainly motivated by the policy goal of cost containment.[33] The first *Health Insurance Cost Containment Act* was enacted in 1976, followed by several other similar laws such as the *Hospital Cost Containment Act* of 1981. Their common feature was a set of instruments aimed primarily at limiting prices and quantities, or shifting costs from the health-insurance funds to other insurance plans (especially sickness insurance) through the exclusion of certain benefits or cost-sharing. In addition, these early laws tried to bring about structural changes in the health-care system in a variety of steps: (i) the attempt to limit spending to the level of revenues received; (ii) the use of prospective budgets to contain spending; (iii) measures to further the transparency of benefits provided by the health-care system, through better use of information or attempts at standardization; (iv) the use of co-insurance with the stated aim of influencing the utilization of services; and (v) rules affecting the contracts between health-insurance funds and providers, largely with the aim of improving efficiency. Although cost-containment measures such as the *Health Reform Act* of 1989 did lead to temporary decreases in expenditures, the underlying trend of growing health costs reasserted itself.

The Structural Health Reform Act of 1993

The economic, social, and political pressures triggered by rising contribution rates led to the passage of the *Structural Health Reform Act* of 1993. The development of this legislation was a typical example of Germany's interlocking federalism and corporatist system. The process of change began with intensive discussions within the self-administration system. A consensus emerged at this level on many of the elements eventually included in the Act; for example, after lengthy debates the necessity of a risk-equalization mechanism for statutory health-insurance plans was generally acknowledged. However, the way in which this mechanism would be organized (nationwide versus regional, for example) had not been agreed to and it was left for the legislative bodies to define.

Because the *Structural Health Reform Act* affected the Länders' budgeting role in the hospital sector, the legislation had to be adopted in both the Bundestag and the Bundesrat. While the Act is a federal law and is legally binding nationwide, its passage was only possible with the agreement of a majority within the Bundesrat. In 1992–93, the liberal/conservative federal government held a majority in the Bundestag, while the Social Democrats who governed a majority of the Länder in various coalitions held a majority in the Bundesrat. The *Structural Reform Act* could, therefore, only be enacted by a coalition of liberals, conservatives, and Social Democrats on the federal level.

In the end, the *Structural Health Reform Act* had two overall strategies. The first strategy focused on short-run measures designed to stabilize the precarious financial position of health-insurance funds and prevent a major increase in contribution rates through massive efforts at cost containment. The second strategy consisted of longer run structural reforms that would prove to be more effective than the more short-term measures of cost containment contemplated by the earlier acts.

To stabilize contribution rates and gain time for longer term measures, the growth in health spending in all major sectors was tied to the growth in revenues (i.e., to the growth of the wage bill). These short-run measures included the following steps for the period from 1993 through 1995: (i) overall budgeting of incomes of ambulatory-care physicians; (ii) budgeting of hospital spending;[34] and (iii) overall budgeting of dentists' incomes, with some exceptions. Additionally, the package included a one-time 10 percent reduction in dentists' remuneration in 1993 for prosthetic and orthopedic measures and a 5 percent reduction for the technical services of dental laboratories; (iv) overall budgeting of spending for pharmaceuticals and for medical and technical aids; (v) a 5 percent reduction in the prices of drugs not yet subject to a fixed-price regimen, and a 2 percent reduction for drugs bought for self-medication; (v) the introduction of co-payments for pharmaceuticals included in the fixed-price regimen, with co-payments varying by package size starting in 1994; and (vi) an increase in co-payment rates in hospitals.

The long-run measures of the *Structural Health Reform Act* focused on structural reforms. Their aim was to remedy the causes rather than the symptoms of expenditure growth. If successful, they should obviate the necessity for a continuing sequence of short-term, cost-containment measures. The long-run measures included:

First, a fundamental change was made in the system of hospital remuneration, beginning in 1996. In place of a system covering costs incurred, individual "prices" were to be paid for specific services or for diagnosis-related overall benefits (similar to DRGs). Second, better coordination or integration of ambulatory and hospital care took place. Hospitals may treat patients on an ambulatory basis before and after the actual period of stay; hospitals were opened for ambulatory operations; joint use of medical technology by hospital and ambulatory-care doctors was encouraged. Third, a change in the division of labour between general practitioners and specialists occurred. This was to be accomplished through a change in the system of remuneration, away from a fee-for-service system toward a more global price system for particular types of services. The major aim was to strengthen the general practitioner and give greater weight to counselling and service activities by providing a flat-rate payment for services.

Attempts to influence the number of doctors and their regional distribution by speciality, in order to provide a curb on the further expansion of the quantity of health goods provided was number four. Fifth, a so-called "positive list" of drugs that are eligible for reimbursement by statutory health-insurance funds was instituted. And finally, organizational reforms to enhance competition among statutory health-insurance funds were set up. By extending the right of choice among different types of statutory health-insurance funds to blue-collar workers, competition among funds was increased significantly. Starting in 1996, all insured persons were able to choose among the major funds. To prevent adverse-selection processes and to maintain the principle of solidarity within a competitive system, a mechanism for equalizing risks among funds was initiated beginning in 1994.

The Risk-Equalization Mechanism

The risk-equalization mechanism within the statutory health insurance system was a central element of the *Structural Reform Act*. This provision had four original goals.[35] The first goal was to strengthen solidarity within the statutory health insurance system by reducing differences in contribution rates. Large variations in contribution rates between funds and between regions conflict with the idea of solidarity, and were considered to be unjust as long as people could not choose freely among different funds. Thus any system of transfers between funds and regions should be designed to reduce differences in contribution rates.

The second goal was to maintain the organizational diversity of the statutory health-insurance system. Large differences in contribution rates endanger the economic survival of funds with rates significantly above the average, especially if the insured can choose freely between funds, as they could beginning in 1996. In the German view, only a vigorous diversity of funds on the local or regional level can ensure effective self-administration and interaction between funds and providers. In light of this goal, any system of transfers between funds and regions should ensure that no fund could increase its attractiveness to employees and employers by harming other funds through risk selection.

The third goal was to establish equal starting conditions for all funds in an increasingly competitive environment, caused by extending the right of choice among different types of statutory health-insurance funds to blue-collar workers. Differences in the socio-economic composition of the insured, such as their age and income structure should not be influenced by the funds. Nevertheless, such differences substantially account for variations in contribution rates. Since competition between funds should concentrate on factors within the direct responsibility of the funds (such as administrative costs[36] and regional differences in the structure and costs of health-providers), the socio-economic influences on costs and contribution rates needed to be mathematically equalized before competition was introduced. Accordingly, a risk-equalization mechanism that accounts for all socio-economic differences influencing contribution rates is an imperative for increasing competition among funds. The objective here is not to eliminate all differences in contribution rates, but to eliminate those differences due to variations in risk structure. When this risk-equalization process is fully implemented, differences in contribution rates are expected primarily to reflect differences in administrative efficiency and supply structures.

The final goal was to reduce the danger that the introduction of more competitive elements within the statutory health-insurance system would lead to risk selection by the funds. While this kind of "skimming" is unlawful — funds are largely required to insure whoever applies for insurance — the US experience shows the high potential for risk selection. By eliminating the higher financial burdens of high-risk groups such as the elderly through a risk-equalization mechanism, active and adverse risk selection becomes less attractive for the funds.

To advance these goals, the *Structural Health Reform Act* of 1993 introduced a risk-equalization mechanism (REM) with the following characteristics.

- The REM basically equalizes the differences in contribution rates that are caused by the following four socio-demographic factors: age, sex, income (the individual health-insurance funds' payroll base), and family size (number of insured dependants).
- Health funds are financially compensated for deviations in their risk structure from the average structure of all statutory funds included in

the equalization mechanism. The basis for the calculation of transfers is the average costs of all health-insurance funds, not the individual expenditures of the fund concerned.

- The REM is calculated within the statutory health-insurance system only, and it therefore involves transfers only among the statutory funds. Neither the private health-insurance sector nor any level of government is financially involved in this mechanism.

- The REM is calculated on a national level.[37] The only exception to this concerns east Germany. Due to the fundamental differences between west and east Germany in socio-economic conditions (especially wages) and the structures of health care, the equalization mechanism is currently calculated separately for both parts of the country. The REM might therefore be defined as "bi-regional" rather than truly national. Since January 1999, the income factor of the REM is calculated on a truly national level, leading to transfers of DM 1.2 billion in 1999 from the west to the east.[38]

- Interregional differences in the income of the insured are compensated for by this mechanism. Since incomes vary significantly among regions, income differences account for much of the transfer within the REM.[39] However, a risk equalization on a national level does not necessarily mean that all funds must, in future, be organized on a national level. Rather, the idea is that contribution rates are calculated on the regional or local level where competition among funds takes place, while national risk equalization reflects the commitment to nationwide solidarity among the insured.[40]

- The equalization mechanism includes all types of funds. This leads to significant transfers among different types of funds, such as from the substitute funds to the general funds.

The risk-equalization mechanism has led to a reduction in contribution rates for the general funds and the guild-based funds, and increases for company-based funds (see Figure 6). While the average contribution rate within the statutory health-insurance system as a whole rose by only 0.01 percentage points between 1993 and 1996, the contribution rates of company-based funds rose by 0.64 percentage points. Due to significant differences in the risk structures among funds, large transfers flowed between them. While the general funds received more than DM 11 billion, the white-collar substitute funds alone paid DM 10.7 billion. The overall range of contribution rates was reduced from

FIGURE 6
Comparing Contribution Rates before (1993) and directly (1996) after the
Introduction of the Risk-Equalization Mechanism

	General Funds	Company-based Funds	Guild-based Funds	Substitute Funds (white-collar workers)	Average of Statutory Health-Insurance Funds
Ø rate in Jan. 1993 (%)	14,07	11,77	13,28	13,19	13,42
Ø rate in Jan. 1996 (%)	13,85	12,41	12,96	13,40	13,43
Range in 1993 (in percentage points)	5,0	8,1	5,2	2,5	9,0
Range in 1996 (in percentage points)	2,3	5,9	2,7	1,1	6,5
Transfers in 1995 (in billion DM)	+11,15	–1,03	–0,27	–10,7	–

Note: "+" signifies received transfers; "–" signifies transfers paid. Not included are the miners' fund (+ 1,872 billion DM) and the substitute funds for blue collar workers (–1,00 billion DM).

Source: Author's compilation based on data from the German Health Ministry.

nine percentage points to 6.5 points. While this reduction certainly was partly a result of transfers caused by the REM, the fusion of many general funds on the state level also added to this effect.

The REM, however, did not eliminate differences in contribution rates among types of funds or states. On the contrary, contribution rates in the city-states of Berlin, Bremen, and Hamburg rose, even though they had already been very high before 1995. While this effect may be a surprise on first sight, it is logical. The average wages in the city-states are above the national average. At the same time, the supply of health care (the number of physicians, the number and equipment of hospitals) is very pronounced and therefore costly. The above-average incomes of these cities are considered in the REM and lead to payments by the city-state funds into the mechanism, but the higher costs they face remain. Hence the increase in contribution rates. This effect, however, is consistent with the goals of the risk-equalization formula, as the supply-side and its costs can, in the long run, be influenced by the funds.

THE CURRENT DEBATE ON REGIONALISM IN THE GERMAN HEALTH-CARE SYSTEM

The debate on the pros and cons of a further regionalization of the German health-care system is as old as the discussion of structural reform to the statutory health-insurance system.[41] However, the financial burdens imposed on certain funds and regions following the introduction of risk equalization has reinforced the debate.

Figure 7 briefly summarizes the main arguments used by both sides in the debate on regionalizing the statutory health-insurance system. Until recently this debate closely followed the lines of self-interest within the self-administering system. It was therefore a debate between those funds that would have to pay into a nationwide risk-equalization mechanism (substitute and company-based funds) against those funds that would benefit from such a mechanism (general funds). It was also a debate between funds organized on a national level, which feared that regional risk equalization might lead to the need for a regional organization (mostly the substitute funds), and funds that already had regional structures (mostly the general funds).

The debate has centred on three issues. The first is whether risk equalization should be organized on a regional or national level. While the discussion has followed along the lines of financial interest, the fundamental, theoretical question is one of a definition of solidarity within statutory health insurance. Are the insured of the statutory health-insurance system a collective risk group, or is the individual type of fund the primary risk group and therefore responsible for its risk structure and its contribution rates? By deciding on nationwide (or rather "bi-regional") risk equalization, the legislature came down on the side of nationwide solidarity, an understanding that is underlined by the introduction of a truly national equalization mechanism for income differences within the health insurance system in 1999.[42] The character of the REM (nationwide versus regional) in itself does not affect the supply-side, since regional and local negotiations between fund associations and provider associations are not altered. Nor does it affect the federal and state governments. The federal

FIGURE 7
Positions on Regionalizing Statutory Health Insurance

Pro Regionalization	*Contra Regionalization*
P1. Providing equal living conditions within Germany (art. 72 GG) does not mean that prices and supply-side structures have to be equal on the national level.	C1. Regionalization leads to a "drifting apart" of supply structures as all contracts, including the general framework, between providers and funds would then be negotiated on a regional basis.
P2. Supply-side differences in quantity and quality are paid for by the "beneficiaries" on the local level.	C2. Regionalizing the statutory health-insurance contradicts the government's goal of narrowing the range of contribution rates.
P3. The health-insurance funds must be able to act, and decide, on a local level, since it is there that health care takes place.	C3. Calculating nationwide contribution rates is in accord with providing equal living conditions within the German federal system (art. 72 GG).
P4. Calculating nationwide contribution rates leads to interregional transfers within funds: regions with low-cost health supplies subsidize regions with expensive, high-quality supply structures.	C4. Further regionalization leads to an increase in administrative costs and to a weakening of the negotiation position of the funds in negotiations between funds and health-care providers.
P5. Having both nationwide and regional contribution rates leads to distortions in the competition between funds — a competition that takes place on the regional level.	C5. Health policy and solidarity do not stop at the borders of the states (Länder).
P6. Regionalization leads to a strengthening of regional responsibilities. State governments are better integrated in these responsibilities (e.g., in hospital-planning).	C6. The current database makes it impossible to regionalize structures at the appropriate local level.
P7. Calculating contribution rates on a regional level increases efficiency in health care.	

Source: Author's compilation based on Dietmar Wassener, *Das Gesundheitsstrukturgesetz 1993 und die Organisationsreform der gesetzlichen Krankenversicherung* (Frankfurt a. M.: Peter Lang Verlag, 1995).

government still determines general guidelines, and the state governments are still responsible for hospital planning.

The second major issue is whether risk equalization should be organized primarily within each type of fund, or also among different types of funds. Here too, the legislature decided that nationwide solidarity means equalizing risks among all funds and not only within the different types of funds.

The third question is whether contribution rates should be calculated on a regional level by all funds.[43] As some funds, especially the substitute funds, calculate nationwide contribution rates, significant sums of money are being transferred between states even without any equalizing mechanisms. For example, while persons insured in Hamburg's funds receive transfers of DM 306 million (DM 172 per capita), the insured in Baden-Württemberg pay DM 334 million (DM 38 per capita).[44] Regionalizing the calculation of contribution rates for all funds by law would therefore reduce inter-state transfers significantly. The main argument for such a regionalization is the principle that since competition takes place on a regional level, prices (i.e., contribution rates) should also be calculated regionally.[45]

The debate on regionalizing certain aspects of the statutory health-insurance system, however, is not a discussion on the principles of political federalism in Germany. Core aspects are never seriously questioned. While risk equalization may take place on a national level, negotiations between fund associations and provider associations are still mostly a regional affair. The prevailing federal principle within the self-administration system is not affected: the pricing framework is still set on a national level, while the actual prices and structures are set at the state level and in the case of hospitals at the local level.

The roles of federal and state governments are not affected by discussions of the ideal structure for the statutory health-insurance system. Whether the risk-equalization mechanism is nationwide or regional, or contribution rates are calculated regionally does not change government roles. The federal government still determines general health-policy guidelines and is only marginally involved financially and state governments are still responsible for hospital planning investments.

While the debate on whether or not contribution rates should be calculated on a regional level focuses on statewide rates, this is only the result of an inadequate database.[46] In theory, if contribution rates are regionalized for all funds, it should be done on a more local level where competition really takes place and a "just" allocation of resources is given.[47]

Debating on a Political Level

The risk-equalization mechanism has a regional aspect, which is shown in Figure 8. While, for example, on average funds in Bavaria, Baden-Württemberg or Hamburg paid substantially into the REM, the health-insurance funds of states such as Niedersachsen or Saarland received significant transfers.[48]

These transfers have to be put into perspective: both Bavaria and Baden-Württemberg are rather large states so that the transfers per insured person in 1995 amounted to only DM 85 and DM 145 respectively (see Figure 8). Nevertheless, these interregional transfers have been criticized not only by those funds that felt the financial burden of risk equalization, but increasingly also by some states whose insured citizens are, on average, net payers into the mechanism. In particular, the governments of Bavaria and Baden-Württemberg criticize the fact that many of "their" citizens provide annual transfers to the insured of other states.[49]

FIGURE 8
Interregional Transfers Caused by the Risk-Equalization Mechanism, 1995

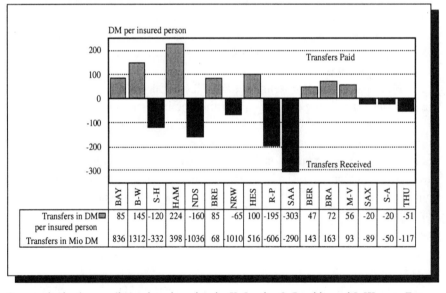

	BAY	B-W	S-H	HAM	NDS	BRE	NRW	HES	R-P	SAA	BER	BRA	M-V	SAX	S-A	THU
Transfers in DM per insured person	85	145	-120	224	-160	85	-65	100	-195	-303	47	72	56	-20	-20	-51
Transfers in Mio DM	836	1312	-332	398	-1036	68	-1010	516	-606	-290	143	163	93	-89	-50	-117

Source: Author's compilation based on data by K. Jacobs, S. Reschke and J. Wasem, *Zur funktionalen Abgrenzung von Bei-tragssatzregionen in der gesetzlichen Krankenversicherung* (Baden-Baden: Nomos, 1998).

The Bavarian government argues that the risk-equalization mechanism should be regionalized on a state level, so that no transfers from the REM flow between states (except transfers caused by the nationwide calculation of contribution rates, especially for the substitute funds). The idea is to "reward a successful state policy rather than to punish it" and to create "a clear definition of responsibility for the states."[50] This argument is based on the false idea that it is the state governments that determine the risk structures within the statutory health-insurance system and that it is the state governments rather than the self-administration partners or the federal government that predominantly influence costs within the health sector. It is undoubtedly true, however, that funds in states such as Bavaria could lower their contribution rates if the REM were regionalized.

The Bavarian demand to regionalize the existing equalization mechanism has to be seen in a broader political perspective.[51] Bavaria and Baden-Württemberg consider their contributions to other transfer systems, especially the horizontal inter-state tax transfer system, to be too high. They argue that the current system of transfers between states does not take into proper account the success of the economic and social policies of different states; both Bavaria and Baden-Württemberg have above-average growth rates in GDP and below-average unemployment rates. Both states are seeking to reduce their contributions to the inter-state tax transfer system.[52] The demand to regionalize structures within the social-security system is therefore just one element in a more general discomfort with the financial burdens of the current tax-transfer systems.[53]

Bavaria, Baden-Württemberg, and Hessen have launched a legal challenge to the existing regulations concerning the inter-state tax transfer system in the federal Supreme Court. However, since the health-care sector is self-administered and the involvement of the states is limited, any legal steps taken against the current organizational structures would have to come from the parties involved, namely the funds. Currently there are no court challenges of the equalization mechanism being calculated on the current national (or rather, "bi-regional") level.[54]

CONCLUSIONS

Although the German health-care system faces continual challenges, especially in the form of rising health costs, it has, until now, been quite successful in meeting them. The German system is far from ideal, but it is widely considered to be highly effective in terms of health outcomes. Reforms of any kind are inevitably accompanied by clashes of interest and discontent for some, but the continual reform of the German health-care system on a largely consensual basis and its ability to reform itself can to a large extent be attributed to its basic structure and underlying principles: solidarity, subsidiarity, and corporatist self-administration.

In the German view, solidarity means that the costs and benefits of health care should be broadly shared among all groups and members of society. At the level of individual funds, this principle is reflected in the calculation of contribution rates according to individual financial ability, while benefits are granted according to need. On the national level, this principle is reflected in the importance given to the idea that a uniformity of living conditions for the whole of Germany should be achieved and maintained. This idea leads to a wide array of transfer systems, including both a horizontal inter-state system of tax transfers and a nationwide risk-equalization mechanism within the statutory health-insurance system that assumes that the relevant risk group consists of all insured persons, no matter in which German state they live. This understanding of solidarity is the bedrock on which all negotiations of health policy changes and structural reforms are based.

The principle of subsidiarity leads to the German view that whatever social aspects can be regulated on a state or regional level should not be delegated to the federal level. This in turn means that the federal government's role in the health-care sector is largely restricted to setting a legal framework. The state governments have little legislative influence in the health-care sector other than through the mechanisms of an interlocking federalism represented by the Bundesrat. Unlike the federal government, however, they do play a direct role in financing the system. By being responsible for hospital planning and financing investment in this sector, they play an active part in day-to-day health policy.

It is important to note, however, that while many structures in the health-care sector reflect the fact that Germany is a federal state, federalism itself is not a constituent element of the German health-care system. Rather, the German view that health care should be organized according to the principle of subsidiarity is the basis for an independent system of non-governmental, self-administered organizations. Subsidiarity within self-administration means that, while the general legislative framework is set on the national level, the actual price negotiations between funds and provider associations take place at the local level in the case of the hospital sector and at the regional level in the case of ambulatory care. Subsidiarity is also reflected in the relative independence of each fund as an institution of risk-sharing. In a way, therefore, subsidiarity counterbalances the nationwide definition of solidarity.

The German health-care system is mostly self-administered. It is employers and employees who administer the different social insurance plans through representatives' assemblies and executive boards at which both employees and employers are equally represented. As far as the health sector is concerned, these legally independent demand-side organizations face equally independent, self-administered, supply-side organizations of physicians and hospitals. Self-administration and subsidiarity lead to the highly decentralized structure of the statutory health-care funds and a relatively small direct influence of both the federal and regional governments. This, in turn, leaves much of the operative level of health policy to self-administration. Together with the general corporatist dimension of the German health-care system, this is reflected in a complex system of cooperation and consensus-seeking mechanisms within the self-administration system, including arbitration committees and the Concerted Action for Health Care.

All in all, the German health-care system can be described as a structure in which a fairly decentralized system of independent providers and demand-side organizations is held together by a federal legislative framework and a common set of undisputed principles.

The general acceptance within German society of basic principles such as solidarity and subsidiarity contributes to the relatively high degree of political consensus and stability within the health-care sector. There are no fundamental, unresolvable disputes over federalizing health policy or privatizing health risks. However, the complexity of the interlocking German federalism and its corporatist structures, especially in the field of social security, does tend to obstruct policy initiatives aimed at the solution of those complex problems that emerge in any welfare state. Reforms that must appease all participants — if they happen at all — are often very slow to come.

In the past, the German health-care system has proven able to adapt to new challenges without sacrificing its principles. In the face of increased financial constraints, however, this ability will be challenged continually and ever more forcefully. Reforming the German health-care system therefore resembles a journey on the narrow road between two options: social stability and a general will to cooperate on one side, and an inability to implement reforms that may be necessary to maintain the popular and effective health-care system on the other.

NOTES

[1]This is only intended to be a very brief introduction to the German federal system. For more detailed information see, for example, Paul Pierson and Stephan Leibfried, "Multitiered Institutions and the Making of Social Policy," in *European Social Policy: Between Fragmentation and Integration*, ed. S. Leibfried and P. Pierson (Washington, DC: The Brookings Institution, 1995); H. Laufer and U. Münch, *Das föderative System der Bundesrepublik Deutschland* (Opladen: UTB, 1998); R. Watts, *Comparing Federal Systems* (Kingston and Montreal: McGill-Queen's University Press for Institute of Intergovernmental Relations, 1996); R.O. Schultze, "Föderalismus," in *Die westlichen Länder*, ed. M.G. Schmidt, Vol. 3 (München, 1992). The following passages rely heavily on Ursula Münch's remarks on German federalism presented at the International Comparative Federalism Workshop on Disability, organized by the Institute of Intergovernmental Relations, Queen's University on 23 September 1998 in Kingston. See U. Münch, "The Governance of Disability Programs in the German Intergovernmental Regime." Paper presented at the International Comparative Federalism Workshop on Disability.

[2]Münch, "The Governance of Disability Programs in the German Intergovernmental Regime."

[3]The aspects of the financial transfers in the German tax system are discussed in Deutsches Institut für Wirtschaftsforschung, "Länderfinanzausgleich: Neuer Verteilungsstreit zwischen Ost und West," *Wochenbericht* 65 (7):133-41 and B. Huber, "Der Finanzausgleich im deutschen Föderalismus," *Aus Politik und Zeitgeschichte* 24:22-30.

[4]Deutsches Institut für Wirtschaftsforschung, "Länderfinanzausgleich."

[5]See R.O. Schultze, "Statt Subsidiarität und Entscheidungsautonomie – Politikverflechtung und kein Ende: Der deutsche Föderalismus nach der Vereinigung," *Staatswissenschaften und Staatspraxis* 4:225-55.

[6]Both vertical and horizontal meetings also take place along party lines, that is, for example, between a Social-Democratic federal government and Social-Democratic state governments on one hand and among different Social-Democratic state governments (the so-called A-Länder) on the other.

[7]F.W. Scharpf, "The Joint Decision Trap: Lessons from German Federalism and European Integration," *Public Administration* 66 (1988):239-78. Ex-Chancellor Helmut Schmidt aptly compared the German system to an oil tanker: once in motion it is very hard to stop and even harder to turn around.

[8]For a practical example of the consensus mechanisms in German social policy, see the discussion of the "making" of the *Structural Health Reform Act* below.

[9]Heinz Lampert, *Lehrbuch der Sozialpolitik*, 3d ed. (Berlin: Springer, 1994).

[10]N. Blüm, "Sozialstaat als Geltungsauftrag," in *Übersicht über die Soziale Sicherheit*, ed. Bundesminister für Arbeit und Sozialordnung, pp. 23-29.

[11]In 1995, a total of DM 1,101 billion were spent on social security. Out of this sum about DM 760 billion (70 percent) were administered by social insurance funds. See Bundesministerium für Arbeit und Sozialordnung (BMA), *Arbeits-und Sozialstatistik. Hauptergebnisse 1997* (Bonn: BMA, 1997).

[12]Deutsches Institut für Wirtschaftsforschung — Economic Consequences of German Unification and its Policy Implications for Korea, Berlin.

[13]J. Wysong and Th. Abel, "Risk Equalization, Competition and Choice: A Preliminary Assessment of the 1993 German Health Care Reforms," *Soziale Präventivmedizin* 41 (1996):213; see also D. Stone, "The Struggle for the Soul of Health Insurance," *Journal of Health Politics, Policy and Law* 18,2 (1993):287-317; and U. Reinhardt, "Accountable Health Care: Is it Compatible with Social Solidarity?" Annual lecture, Office of Health Economics, London, 1997.

[14]The fifth volume of the Social Code (*Sozialgesetzbuch*) is the basis for all regulations concerning the health-care sector.

[15]M. Schneider, "Evaluation of Cost-Containment Acts in Germany," in *Health: Quality and Choice*, Health Policy Studies No. 4 (Paris: OECD, 1994), pp. 63-81.

[16]The city of Hamburg is one of the 15 German states. The other so-called "city-states" (*Stadtstaaten*) are Bremen and Berlin.

[17]Dietmar Wassener, "Krankenversicherungsschutz," in *Gesundheitsbericht für Deutschland*, ed. Statistisches Bundesamt (Stuttgart, 1998), pp. 26-30.

[18]D. Leopold, "Die Organisationsreform bei den Krankenkassen schreiten voran," *Die Beiträge zur Sozial- und Arbeitslosenversicherung* 8/9 (1995):10-16.

[19]As the miners' sickness fund, the seamen's sickness fund, and the agricultural sickness funds have rather small market shares, they are not included with this discussion.

[20]For a discussion of market shares, see Wassener, "Krankenversicherungsschutz."

[21]Dietmar Wassener, *Das Gesundheitsstrukturgesetz 1993 und die Organisationsreform der gesetzlichen Krankenversicherung* (Frankfurt a. M.: Peter Lang Verlag, 1995).

[22]Organisation for Economic Co-operation and Development (OECD), *Financing and Delivering Health Care: A Comparative Analysis of OECD Countries* (Paris: OECD, 1987).

[23]In general, health benefits are provided in the form of real benefits. Nevertheless, as Figure 3 indicates, direct cash benefits such as sick pay account for about one-quarter of total expenditures.

[24]W. Müller, "Ausgaben für Gesundheit 1996," *Soziale Sicherheit* 47,11 (1998):915-23.

[25]In general sick pay is paid by the employer for the first six weeks of any illness (about DM 58 billion in 1996). Any further sick pay is then paid by the health-insurance funds (about DM 54 billion in 1996).

[26]*Sachverständigenrat für die Konzertierte Aktion im Gesundheitswesen — Das Gesundheitswesen im vereinten Deutschland.* Jahresgutachten, 1991 (Baden-Baden: Nomos, 1991).

[27]R.J. Blendon and J.M. Blendon *et al.*, "Who Has the Best Health Care System?" *Health Affairs* 14,4 (1995):220-43.

[28]Bundesministerium für Gesundheit — Argumentationspapier (BMG). *Entwurf eines Gesetzes der Fraktionen SPD und Bündnis 90/Die Grünen zur Stärkung der Solidarität in der gesetzlichen Krankenversicherung — GKV — Solidaritätsstärkungsgesetz* (Bonn: BMG, 1998).

[29]Organisation for Economic Co-operation and Development (OECD), *OECD Health Data 1997* (Paris: OECD, 1998); G. Schieber, J.-P. Poullier and L. Greenwald, "U.S. Health Expenditure Performance: An International Comparison and Data Update," *Health Care Financing Review* 13,4 (1992):1-15; and R. Saltman, "Analyzing the Evidence on European Health Care Reforms," *Health Affairs* 17,2 (1998):85-107.

[30]As pointed out above, contributions are calculated as a percentage of gross wages up to a nationally defined income ceiling. This ceiling determines the maximum contribution and is adjusted if average incomes rise.

[31]Bundesministerium für Gesundheit (BMG), *Die Gesetzliche Krankenversicherung im Jahr 1995* (Bonn: BMG, 1996).

[32]This issue had led policymakers and researchers to focus on why expenditures and contribution rates vary systematically between regions, and between and within various types of funds. Regional variations in physician's practice patterns, in hospital costs, and in utilization rates certainly account for some of these differences. Differences in efficiency in the administration of the various funds is also cited as an important source of variations in expenditure and contribution rates.

[33]The description of German health-care policy goals is based on M. Pfaff, "Health Policy Formulation and the Role of Information in Managing Change: A German Perspective." Paper presented at the Four Country Conference on Health Reform, Health Policy — Towards 2000, Montebello, Quebec, 16–18 May 1996. See also B. Abel-Smith and E. Mossialos, "Cost Containment and Health Care Reform: A Study of the European Union," *Health Policy* 28 (1994):89-132.

[34]However, due to a list of clauses allowing for exceptions or addenda to these budgets such as added employment of personnel, higher growth in salaries of said personnel, higher growth in the number of mid-wives, and improvement in psychiatric care etc. — hospital spending grew much more than the wage bill.

[35]Wassener, *Das Gesundheitsstrukturgesetz 1993*.

[36]Administrative costs account for about 5 percent of total costs within statutory health insurance.

[37]The reference for all calculations are therefore national, and not regional, averages within statutory health insurance.

[38]See S. Dudey, K. Jacbos and S. Reschke, *Auf dem Weg zu einem ungeteilten gesamtdeutschen: Konzeptionelle Grundlagen und empirische Konsequenzen möglicher regelungsgebundener Übergangsmodelle* (Berlin, 1999). The introduction of a truly national REM (equalizing not only income-differences but age, sex, and family size as well) is proposed by some east German Länder (e.g., Brandenburg) and is currently the focus of discussion between local and substitute funds.

[39]While, for example, in 1995 the relevant average annual gross income of general fund members was DM 40,964 in Baden-Württemberg, it was DM 36,413 in Niedersachsen, and only DM 28,703 in Saxony (see Bundesministerium für Gesundheit, *Die Gesetzliche Krankenversicherung im Jahr 1995*).

[40]Dietmar Wassener, "Auswirkungen Bundesweiter und Regionaler Risikostrukturausgleiche," in *Wahlfreiheit und Solidarität*, ed. AOK-Bundesverband (Bonn, 1992), pp. 55-66.

[41]See, for example, P. Biene-Dietrich, "Regionale Aspekte einer Organisationsreform der Gesetzlichen Krankenversicherung," in *Wahlfreiheit und Solidarität*, ed. AOK-Bundesverband (Bonn, 1992), pp. 67-72; K. Jacobs, "Anforderungen an die gesetzliche Krankenversicherung zur Verbesse-rung der regionalen Angebots- und Nachfragestrukturen im Gesundheitswesen," *Informationen zur Raumentwicklung* 2,3 (1990):119-27. K. Kirschner, "Regionalität versus Zentralismus," *Arbeit und Sozialpolitik* 46,3-4 (1992):4-8; and G. Schmidbauer, "Spielräume und Einschränkungen für eine regional orienerte Gesundheitspolitik," *Information zurRaumentwicklung* 3,4 (1985):187-93 among others.

[42]While the old conservative/liberal federal government confined this mechanism to the years 1999 to 2001, the new Social-Democrat/Green federal government cancelled this time limitation.

[43]Note that regionalizing the calculation of contribution rates neither means that the equalization mechanism would have to be regional too, nor does it necessarily mean that all funds would need to be organized totally on a regional level (i.e., splitting up the nationwide substitute funds)!

[44]See K. Jacobs, S. Reschke and J. Wasem, *Zur funktionalen Abgrenzung von Bei-tragssatzregionen in der gesetzlichen Krankenversicherung* (Baden-Baden: Nomos, 1998).

[45]D. Pfeiffer, "Regionalisierung und (k)ein Ende," *Die Ersatzkasse* 52,1 (1998):33-36.

[46]Most data on cost, supply and demand structures are only (if at all) available on a state level.

[47]See, for example, M. Pfaff and D. Wassener, "Die Bedeutung des Risikostrukturausgleichs für den Kassenwettbewerb und die solidarische Wettbewerbsordnung," in *Fairneß, Effizienz und Qualität in der Gesundheitsversorgung*, ed. Gesellschaft für Recht und Politik im Gesundheitswesen (Berlin: Springer, 1998), pp. 9-21; and E. Wille and M. Schneider, "Zur Regionalisierung in der gesetzlichen Krankenversicherung," in *Fairneß, Effizienz und Qualität in der Gesundheitsversorgung*, ed. Gesellschaft für Recht und Politik im Gesundheitswesen (Berlin: Springer, 1998), pp. 23-58.

[48]The transfers discussed here are the net sums of transfers paid or received in the different states. Within the states some individual funds may have received transfers while others paid.

[49]See B. Stamm, "Wettbewerbsföderalismus in der Sozialversicherung," *Soziale Sicherheit* 47,1 (1998):1-3.

[50]Ibid., p. 3.

[51]This demand is supported by Baden-Württemberg and, as it seems, to some extent by Saxony.

[52]Deutsches Institut für Wirtschaftsforschung, "Länderfinanzausgleich."

[53]Bavaria not only wants the REM to be regionalized but also puts forward a regionalized calculation of contribution rates to the unemployment and pension insurance.

[54]There is, however, court action against the risk-equalization mechanism in general, although it is basically about the socio-economic factors included in the REM.

4

AUSTRALIAN INTERGOVERNMENTAL RELATIONS AND HEALTH

Linda Hancock

INTRODUCTION

Health is high on the political agenda in Australia. As an area of concurrent responsibility, shared between the Commonwealth and state governments and between public and private providers, health policy is both politically sensitive and practically challenging, an area fraught with ongoing demands at all stakeholder levels. Recurring themes in federal-state relations are concerns about funding, and the battle between the Commonwealth's desire for cohesive national policies on the one hand and the states' desire for greater discretion and flexibility on the other.

This chapter is divided into five sections. The first provides a brief description of the Australian health-care system, and the second gives an overview of the basic characteristics of Australian federalism. The third section then analyzes the intersection of federalism and the Australian health-care system, highlighting federal practices, funding mechanisms and institutional arrangements, and assessing the impact of federalism on health-care provision in Australia. The fourth section canvasses four issues that highlight the volatility of federal-state relations in health: rising health-care costs; shifts in the private/public mix of health care; controversies over "tied" Commonwealth-state grants; and the ambiguities of duplication and cost-shifting between levels of government. A brief final section then pulls together the primary conclusions.

The Australian Health System

Medicare, the national health scheme established in 1984, provides universal access to free medical, pharmaceutical, and public hospital care. The Commonwealth government provides for nursing homes and access to doctors and pharmaceuticals under the Medical Benefits and Pharmaceutical Benefits Schemes, which are administered by the federal Health Insurance Commission. Universal access to free public hospital care is established through bilateral Commonwealth-state agreements, negotiated every five years. These agreements provide that treatment beyond these public services — such as private hospital care, dental services treatment, and treatment by other health-care professionals — is paid for by users, either directly or with the assistance of optional private health insurance. Unlike some European countries, Australia does not have a national social insurance scheme based on work-related contributions. Social-security benefits and pensions for the elderly, the unemployed, single parents, and so on are paid by the Commonwealth government out of general revenue. In the case of health, only about 8 percent of health expenditure flows from a special levy on income known as the Medicare Levy; the remainder of the government contribution to health-care costs comes from a mix of federal and state general revenues.

The Australian health-care system is built on the following foundations: (i) the Medicare principles: universal coverage, bulk billing,[1] free access to public hospital care, access to the doctor of choice for out-of-hospital care, and the general freedom of doctors — within accepted clinical practices — to identify appropriate treatment for their patients; (ii) an overarching agreement between the Commonwealth and the states and territories on the principles and framework governing federal-state relations in the health and community services fields; and (iii) under the broad leadership of the Commonwealth, the joint setting of priorities, goals, and quality outcomes for both tiers of government, with the states and territories having increased responsibility for the delivery of services to meet agreed outcomes.

In the Australian context, "health care" includes medical and pharmaceutical services, institutions such as hospitals, nursing homes and ambulances, medical aids and appliances, non-institutional services such as community services and health, dental services, and health research.[2] However, three major items dominate health expenditures and have, in turn, dominated policy reform debates: institutions (about 46 percent of expenditures); medical services (20 percent); and pharmaceuticals (12 percent). Since funding for hospitals is capped and regulated by intergovernmental agreements, rising expenditures on medical services and pharmaceuticals are the focus of reform efforts, even though many argue that more spent upstream on public health would reduce the downstream costs in terms of expensive hospital and medical services.[3]

The response to pressures on the health-care system is shaped by a political context in which governments are advancing a neo-liberal policy agenda. This agenda, which reflects a broad international trend, includes: smaller government and a preference for market mechanisms in the provision of public services; a leaning toward private for-profit rather than public providers; and a business-like management of public agencies through devolution, shifting risk management onto individuals, output-based funding, and performance incentives. In health, this is exemplified by recent policy trends, including budget cuts, rebates for private health insurance in preference to grants to public hospitals, government withdrawal from areas such as dental services, and shifts from government to private sector provision of services through privatization, contracting-out, and reductions in the size of government bureaucracies.

This new political agenda has important implications for intergovernmental relations in the health sector. High on the intergovernmental agenda have been more cohesive national policies and improved efficiency, especially between levels of government. Before turning to those issues, however, it is important to examine the formal parameters for intergovernmental relations set by the Constitution of the country.

AUSTRALIAN FEDERALISM: THE CONSTITUTION

Australian federalism and the principle of power-sharing between federal and state governments is written into the Australian Constitution of 1901, and federalism is based on a constitutional division of powers between two spheres of government: the Commonwealth and state/territory[4] governments. A third sphere, local government, is set up under state constitutions and laws.[5] Described by Emy and Hughes as "a perennial source of tension and debate in Australian politics," federation, they say, was a "pragmatic compromise between the need to cede just enough power to the centre to create a viable Commonwealth government, while leaving the States with sufficient responsibilities for them to agree to join the new union."[6] The founders of Australian federalism intended it would preserve a regional form of government in which states are free to pursue their own policies and the Commonwealth acts "where national interest requires national uniformity."[7] However, the distinctive feature of Australian federalism is the role of concurrent jurisdiction. Galligan argues that rather than separate and distinct governments with separate jurisdictions and policy responsibilities, the "basic principle of design is concurrency, with the Commonwealth and the States having, for the most part, shared roles and responsibilities in major policy and fiscal areas," with overlap and duplication "grounded in the underlying Constitutional system."[8] In the words of an advisory committee, "by world standards, Australian federalism exhibits a very high degree of concurrence."[9]

Given that very few powers are held exclusively by the Commonwealth government, Australian federalism does not reflect a simple hierarchical model. Formal jurisdiction and financial arrangements lead to complex interdependence of the two levels of government. Section 51 of the Constitution of Australia sets out Commonwealth powers, listing 40 heads of power with respect to which the Commonwealth Parliament may pass legislation, and specifies that Commonwealth legislation is paramount in these areas. That is to say, the Commonwealth exercises power concurrently with the states, but Commonwealth law prevails in instances of conflict with state laws. Amendments to the Constitution in 1946 extended the Commonwealth's powers to include laws on pharmaceutical, sickness and hospital benefits, and medical and dental services; and the Commonwealth operates the Medical Benefits and Pharmaceutical Benefits Scheme under the universal Medicare scheme introduced in 1984.

On the financial side, section 96 permits the Commonwealth to give grants to the states on its own terms and conditions: "the Parliament may grant financial assistance to any State on such terms and conditions as the Parliament sees fit." This section takes on particular importance because of the fiscal dominance of the Commonwealth government. Although the Commonwealth's taxation power is a concurrent power under section 51 (ii) of the Constitution, the Commonwealth took over the levying of personal income tax during World War II and a uniform tax scheme came into effect in 1942. After 1946, the Commonwealth decided to continue uniform taxation and to make tax reimbursement grants to the states, a practice that continues to the present day. The Commonwealth's postwar monopoly of income taxation, as well as recent High Court decisions preventing the states from imposing certain taxes on goods,[10] have left the states with a narrow revenue base, and contributed to a large vertical fiscal imbalance. This fiscal reality has been a central feature of Australian federalism. As the Commonwealth-State Relations Committee noted, "the States' role in shaping policy as equal participants in the federation is undermined by the Commonwealth's fiscal dominance."[11] This pattern was shaken up to some extent in July 2000 by the introduction of the Goods and Services Tax (GST), which is discussed further below. But in general, funding transfers from the Commonwealth to the states remain a central focus of much intergovernmental activity and conflict within Australian federalism.

HEALTH AND COMMONWEALTH-STATE RELATIONS: FUNDING AND INSTITUTIONS

With shared or concurrent powers over health matters under the Constitution, attempts to divide responsibility for health-care policy and service delivery between the Commonwealth and the states have been contested. Responsibilities for funding, service provision, and policy direction are the main focus of intergovernmental tensions. There have been some attempts at a clearer division of responsibility but, as Duckett observes, responsibility is not shared in a coherent or consistent manner, and comprehensive national policies are difficult to achieve.[12]

Despite this intergovernmental complexity, the Commonwealth government plays a central role in defining policy. The Commonwealth sets national policy parameters such as medical fees, health insurance rebates, and fees for private patients in public hospitals.[13] In addition to setting the basic parameters of the Medicare Scheme, the Commonwealth has led the joint development of influential national policies, including the National Health Strategy, the National Mental Health Strategy, the National Women's Health Strategy, and the National Disability Strategy, as well as the definition of national standards for institutions such as nursing homes and a common model of hospital funding (the Casemix model), which has now been implemented in various forms by all states and territories. The National Mental Health strategy illustrates this national approach in which the Commonwealth and state governments develop an agreed policy framework. The second National Mental Health Plan (1998–2003) provides an agreed framework for mental health reform identifying three broad themes: promotion and prevention, partnerships in service reform and delivery, and quality and effectiveness. The plan is financed by dedicated funding in the amount of $300 million for mental health services, of which $250 million is allocated broadly on a per capita basis and $50 million is reserved for targeted reforms.[14]

In addition, the Commonwealth has been the driving force propelling the states into greater cooperation around nationally set agendas aimed at microeconomic reform, principally through the Council of Australian

Governments and the National Competition Policy. Although these initiatives are aimed at the whole range of government programs, they have powerful implications for health care, as is discussed more fully below. As Duckett observes: "The Commonwealth government's domination of health policy in Australia prevails despite the fact that its formal constitutional powers with respect to hospitals are limited."[15]

As Tables 1 and 2 show, health is funded from a variety of sources: the Commonwealth, the states, health insurance, and user payments or "out-of-pocket expenses." Government pays for about two-thirds of total health services expenditure, but unpacking the mix of Commonwealth/state/local government funding in health is a challenge for intergovernmental analysts. Actual expenditure figures mask the source of funds, since the Commonwealth government is the major funder of Australian health-care services, as would be expected in light of its monopoly on income tax collection. The states and local governments, however, are the most important providers; they deliver services on the basis of Commonwealth grants directed to them for specific purposes such as hospitals, as well as their own revenue sources. Focusing on the point of expenditure, the Commonwealth government directly funds around 46 percent of recurrent health expenditure; state and local governments fund around 24 percent (although some of this funding comes from Commonwealth grants paid through the states[16]); and the non-governmental sector, including health insurance voluntary private contributor schemes and individuals, through service charges, funds around 31 percent.[17]

COMMONWEALTH-STATE TRANSFERS

Arrangements exist within the federal system for the collection of revenue and the transfer of funds between governments, principally as grants. Australia has been characterized by "the largest degree of vertical fiscal imbalance between its tiers of government of any federal nation."[18] The federal government raised about 73 percent of combined Commonwealth-state government general revenues but its expenditures for its own direct programs were only 58 percent of total general government outlays.[19] Income tax is by far the most important source of Commonwealth revenue. The states rely on Commonwealth grants for about 46 percent of their revenue and raise the balance themselves principally through property, gambling, and business taxes, since they are not permitted to levy income tax or, more recently, excise duties (taxes on the manufacture, distribution and sale of goods).

TABLE 1
Government and Non-Government Sector Expenditure, Current Prices, as a Proportion of Total Health Services Expenditure, 1989–90 to 1997–98 (%)

Year	Government Sector			Non-government Sector[a]	Total Health Services Expenditure
	Commonwealth[a]	State and Local	Total		
1989–90	42.2	26.1	68.3	31.7	100
1990–91	42.2	25.5	67.7	32.3	100
1991–92	42.8	24.6	67.4	32.6	100
1992–93	43.7	23.4	67.1	32.9	100
1993–94	45.3	21.4	66.7	33.3	100
1994–95	45.0	21.7	66.7	33.3	100
1995–96	45.6	22.2	67.7	32.3	100
1996–97	44.8	22.5	67.2	32.8	100
1997–98[b]	45.5	23.6	69.1	30.9	100

Notes: [a]Expenditure by the Commonwealth government and the non-government sector has been adjusted for tax expenditures (see Table 7 of source for health services tax expenditure).
[b]Based on preliminary AIHW and ABS estimates.

Source: AIHW health expenditure database. Australian Institute of Health and Welfare, *Health Expenditure Bulletin No. 15: Australia's Health Services Expenditures to 1997–98* Canberra: AIHW, 1999), p. 5.

TABLE 2
Total Health Services Expenditure, Current Prices, by Area of Expenditure and Source of Funds, 1996–1997 ($ million)

Area of Expenditure	Government Sector			Non-government Sector				Total Expenditure
	Common-wealth	State and Local	Total	Health Insurance Funds	Indivi-duals	Other[b]	Total	
Total hospitals	5,758	5,870	11,628	2,797	384	1,025	4,206	15,834
Recognized public hospitals	5,379	5,541	10,920	360	88	606	1,053	11,973
Private hospitals	354	-	354	2,437	288	415	3,139	3,493
Repatriation hospitals	16	-	16	-	-	-	1	16
Private psychiatric hospitals	9	329	338	-	9	5	13	352
Nursing homes	2,298	156	2,454	-	695	-	695	3,148
Ambulance	46	210	256	93	126	33	252	509
Other institutional (necessary)	-	-	-	-	-	-	-	-
Medical services	6,713	-	6,713	229	818	438	1,485	8,198
Other professional services	203	-	203	225	788	191	1,204	1,407
Total pharmaceuticals	2,718	11	2,729	44	2,245	37	2,327	5,056
Benefit paid pharmaceuticals	2,718	-	2,718	-	550	-	550	3,268
All other pharmaceutical services	-	11	11	44	1,696	37	1,777	1,788
Aids and appliances	154	-	154	184	467	37	688	842

Other non-institutional services	1,246	1,981	3,227	1,128	1,551	12	2,691	5,918
Community and public health[c]	728	1,365	2,093	1	—	3	4	2,097
Dental services	97	297	394	596	1,551	9	2,157	2,551
Administration	421	319	740	530	—	—	530	1,271
Research	462	102	565	—	—	119	119	683
Total non-institutional	11,496	2,095	13,591	1,810	5,870	834	8,514	22,105
Total recurrent expenditure	19,598	8,331	27,929	4,700	7,075	1,892	13,667	41,596
Capital expenditure	58	1,122	1,180	n/a	n/a	n/a	[d]972	2,152
Capital consumption	25	506	531	..	..	..	[e]..	531
Total health expenditure	19,681	9,959	29,640	n/a	n/a	n/a	14,639	44,279

Notes: [a]This table shows the funding provided by the Commonwealth government, state, and territory governments and local government authorities and by the major sources of non-government funding. It does not show gross outlays on health services by the different levels of government or by non-governmental service providers.
[b]"Other" includes expenditure on health services by workers' compensation and compulsory motor vehicle third-party insurers as well as other sources of income (e.g., interest earned) of service providers.
[c]Includes expenditure that was previously classified as "other non-institutional" as well as expenditure on community and public health services.
[d]Capital outlays for the non-governmental sector cannot be allocated according to source funds.
[e]Non-governmental capital consumption (depreciation) expenditure is included as part of recurrent expenditure.

Source: Australian Institute of Health and Welfare, *Health Expenditure Bulletin No. 15*, p. 38.

In the past, payments from the Commonwealth to the states and territories were made principally as either General Revenue Assistance (GRA) or Special Purpose Payments (SPPs).[20] Grants made under GRA were unconditional; they constituted 51 percent of total net Commonwealth transfers to the states (1999–2000) and comprised mainly Financial Assistance Grants (or FAGs). These have largely been replaced in 2000–2001 and 2001–02 by revenue from the GST reform package. Revenues raised by the states can be spent by the states according to their own budget priorities. In contrast, SPPs, of which there are over 100, are subject to conditions reflecting Commonwealth policy objectives or national policy objectives agreed between the Commonwealth and the states. These comprised 49 percent of total net Commonwealth transfers to the states in 1999–2000, but declined to 40.2 percent in the 2001–02 budget.[21] Prior to the GST, GRA and SPPs were the predominant mechanisms for overcoming not only vertical fiscal imbalance but also the horizontal fiscal imbalance resulting from variations in revenue-raising capacities of different states and differences in the costs of providing goods and services across the country. GRA comprised payments to the states which were distributed on the basis of principles applied by the Commonwealth Grants Commission. FAGs accounted for 97 percent of general revenue assistance.[22] Horizontal fiscal equalization principles were embodied in the FAGs in the form of per capita relativities recommended by the Commonwealth Grants Commission with the aim of improving equity for all Australians.[23]

Because of the open-ended nature of some of its programs, especially in the social policy area, the Commonwealth has increased its own outlays at a greater rate than its assistance to the states, and gross assistance to the states has declined overall from 34 percent of Commonwealth outlays in 1976–77 to 27 percent in 1997–98.[24] The declining Commonwealth funding base is a source of persistent complaint from the states. Under the new tax system, GST revenue comprises 53.6 percent of Commonwealth payments to the states, General Assistance 6.2 percent (residue of the previous GRA grants), and SPPs 40.2 percent.[25] GST revenue is predicted to increase the pool of funds available to states. This is still open to speculation.

SPPs come in two forms. Payments from the Commonwealth "through" the states (about one-quarter of SPPs or 12 percent of total Commonwealth payments to the states) are payments that are simply passed onto other bodies such as higher education, university research, non-governmental schools, and local government.[26] In such cases, the states act as agents for the Commonwealth, carrying out what are essentially Commonwealth government programs that, for constitutional reasons, the Commonwealth must fund via the states. In contrast, payments "to" the states (about three-quarters of SPPs or 37 percent of total Commonwealth payments to the states) fund programs administered at the state level. These include hospitals, government schools, aged and disability services, housing, highways, and legal aid. Health-care grants made under the Australian Health Care Agreements make up about half the payments "to" the states.

For the funding year 1999–2000, 12 of the 120 SPPs related directly to health. Table 3 shows the distribution of Commonwealth funding for health as direct Commonwealth expenditure (48 percent), taxation expenditure (1 percent) and SPPs to other levels of government (17 percent) as a percentage of

TABLE 3
Government Sector Funding of Health Services, Current Prices, by Type of Funding, 1989–90 to 1997–98 ($ million)

| Year | Government Sector | | | Net State and Local Government Expenditure[b] | Total Government Sector |
	Direct Expenditure[a]	Taxation Expenditure	SPPs to Other Levels of Government		
1989–90	8,551	61	3,553	7,513	19,677
1990–91	9,288	85	3,827	7,958	21,158
1991–92	10,065	82	4,020	8,138	22,305
1992–93	10,920	91	4,262	8,202	23,494
1993–94	11,763	95	4,808	7,868	24,550
1994–95	12,391	91	4,068	8,460	26,010
1995–96	13,670	141	4,222	9,260	28,293
1996–97	14,333	137	5,348	9,959	29,777
1997–98[c]	15,595	[d]350	5,543	11,159	32,647

Notes: [a]Direct expenditures by the Commonwealth refers to all types of payments made by the Commonwealth government that are *not SPPs* to or for the states and territories.
[b]Net expenditure is total outlays by state and territory governments and by local government authorities *net of revenue and SPPs*.
[c]Based on preliminary AIH and ABS estimates.
[d]$182 million of general health tax rebates and $167 million of PHIIS tax rebates.
Sources: AHIW health expenditure database. (AHIW, *Health Expenditure Bulletin No. 5*, p. 6).

total government funding in 1997–98.[27] The table also shows that the states' own funding accounted for 34 percent of government funding of health services.

Most SPPs are "tied" grants that are subject to conditions, reflecting Commonwealth policy objectives or national policy objectives agreed to by the Commonwealth and the states. Although the conditions differ between programs, and some of the accountability mechanisms for the states' spending appear to be weak, in general SPPs are seen as a means for the Commonwealth to pursue its policy objectives in areas where the states are the primary service providers.

Despite the fact that section 96 grants give the Commonwealth powers to make grants to the states on its own terms and conditions, SPPs remain controversial from the states' points of view. Conditions attached to SPPs can limit the ability of state governments to set their own spending priorities. Furthermore, the ability of states to switch "tied" grants to other purposes is limited because a substantial proportion of SPP funding is for programs in which the Commonwealth exerts either direct control or imposes substantial conditions. Health grants are paid as SPPs, although this has not always been the case. Conditions include general policy requirements such as that states provide free public hospital treatment to Medicare patients as a condition of receiving grants. However, a major point of weakness in health-care funding is the lack of accountability for state's spending under Medicare and Australian Health Care Agreements, a point discussed further in the final section.

The two political parties that dominate Australian politics have differed in their approach to federalism. As a result, the role of SPPs has varied over time, with Labor governments generally favouring tied grants and Liberal/National Party coalitions reducing reliance on them. Tied grants increased during the Whitlam Labor government from 25.8 percent of Commonwealth transfers to the states in 1972–73 to 48.5 percent in 1975–76. Under the Fraser Liberal government, they fell to 41.5 percent in 1980–81 and to 32.7 percent in 1981–82, but they grew again under the Hawke/Keating Labor governments to 52.8 percent in 1995–96. SPPs were reduced under the Howard coalition to 50 percent in 1998–99, fell to around 49 percent of total Commonwealth payments to states in 1999–2000, and to 40.2 percent in the 2000–01 budget.[28] The structuring of health grants as either part of general revenue to the states or as SPPs helps explain a large measure of the variations in the role of SPPs over the last 25 years. Moves were made in the Council of Australian Governments in 1995 and 1996 to untie funds and to "broadband" previously separately funded programs into one payment, obliging states to meet Commonwealth objectives or outcomes but giving them discretion over the means to do so. In recent years, states have put pressure on the Commonwealth to reduce further the proportion of tied grants. However, at the 1999 Premier's Conference, the Commonwealth indicated that it had no intention of further reducing aggregate SPPs as part of the reform agenda outlined under the 1999 Intergovernmental Agreement on the Reform of Commonwealth-State Financial Relations.

Federal-state financial relations are, however, being transformed by the broader process of tax reform, which has been designed to enhance Australia's international competitiveness and encourage new and competitive industries. Excise duties, covered by section 90 of the Constitution, have been interpreted to include broad-based consumption or general sales taxes, which allowed the Commonwealth to introduce the controversial GST. The Howard government's tax package established the GST on goods and services with exemptions for education, health, and some health-related products and, as added in controversial amendments, an exemption for certain items of food. This tax reform has been described as the biggest change in federal-state relations in Australia's history. The tax is to be collected by the Commonwealth and paid to the states after deduction of the costs of collection. Revenue from the GST will replace General Revenue Assistance and some specified state taxes (including wholesale tax, bed taxes, FID and the debit tax).[29]

Whether or not states will be better off under the new tax package is unclear. Some argue that vertical fiscal imbalance will actually be worse than under the previous system, given the exemptions for food, and that political opposition to the GST may lead a future Labor government to take steps that reduce GST revenues. Not surprisingly, some states are now vocal in arguing that a GST will be inadequate in rectifying vertical fiscal imbalance, since it may result both in less income and in less leverage with the Commonwealth. In the past, Premiers' Conferences have been a forum for states' demands for increases in GRA. Replacing such funding with GST revenues based on states' proportionate GST earnings may largely preclude traditional haggling over general funds. States have argued that they lack the broad revenue base needed to respond flexibly to rising service delivery demands and that their reliance on other revenue sources, such as taxes on business and gambling, may be counter-productive for investment and growth or possibly for equity.[30] In addition, some states, such as Victoria, have eroded their traditional revenue base by selling off state-owned enterprises under privatization agendas. These changes do not augur well for states' faith that they have an adequate revenue base to deliver on national and state priorities.

INSTITUTIONAL ARRANGEMENTS: NEW FEDERALISM AND THE COUNCIL OF AUSTRALIAN GOVERNMENTS

The distribution of powers between levels of governments in a federal system and the degree of separateness or independence of the regional level in such systems remain highly charged issues open to change and interpretation. The Constitution established two powerful federal institutions to deal with these issues: the Inter-State Commission (inoperative for most of federation) and the Senate or upper house of the Commonwealth Parliament.[31] In practice, however, neither has provided a forum for mediating between Commonwealth and state governments, and it is therefore important to focus on other more influential intergovernmental institutions.

Historically, Premiers' Conferences have been the main vehicle for determining the amount and distribution of general revenue assistance to the states. These conferences have frequently highlighted states' claims about the negative impact of vertical fiscal imbalance and the need for more funds to flow in an untied form to the states. Other mechanisms for intergovernmental cooperation include Commonwealth-State Ministerial Councils, the Council of Australian Governments (COAG), the Loans Council, and the Treaties Council, along with ministerial conferences in specific policy areas, officials' committees, and bilateral communications government agencies.

By far the most important driving force for national and intergovernmental reform has been COAG. This organization emerged out of the joint review of Commonwealth-state financial arrangements conducted by the Special Premiers' Conference in 1991, under Prime Minister Hawke's "New Federalism" policy.[32] COAG was established in 1992 as an ongoing council. It comprises the prime minister, the premiers and chief ministers and the president of the local government association; and it needs to be understood as a reflection of the concurrent nature of Australian federalism and as evidence of "cooperative federalism in Australia."[33] The New Federalism policy and the continuing role of COAG constituted a means of coordinating intergovernmental arrangements. During the 1990s, the policy prompted both a review of the distribution of taxation powers to reduce vertical fiscal imbalance, and an attempt to provide a clearer definition of roles and responsibilities of governments in program and service delivery. It also entailed a commitment to downscale the trend to increased reliance on tied grants (SPPs).[34]

The New Federalism initiative was in tune with later reforms under the National Competition Policy, which was designed to increase national efficiency and international competitiveness, and to move Australia toward a single national economy. COAG has played a central role in bringing about state-Commonwealth agreement on the National Competition Policy, which in turn has profoundly shaped intergovernmental arrangements across a range of areas, including health. This national reform agenda has involved structural reform of public monopolies, competitive neutrality between public and private sectors, and oversight of prices charged by utilities with monopoly power. Reports congruent with the agenda included the 1996 Industry Commission Inquiry into compulsory competitive tendering, which recommended greater use of contracting-out and compulsory competitive tendering. The intention is to subject a range of sectors to international and domestic competition. This national agenda has important implications for federalism. State governments have been given some discretion as to how they implement the plan, and various state governments have taken a practical approach to implementation in order to minimize adverse regional impacts. Nevertheless, the National Competition Policy is clearly aimed at an integrated national economic policy and more consistent business regulation across the country. Critics warn of the tensions between its agenda of harmonization, uniformity, and decreased regulation on the one hand, and pressures for local diversity and increased regulation on the other.[35]

Building on the Hilmer Report (1993) in April 1995, the Commonwealth, state and territory governments endorsed three intergovernmental agreements relating to National Competition Policy.[36] Governments signed the Competition Code Agreement, the Competition Principles Agreement, and the Implementation and Funding Agreement. These committed governments to implementing significant reforms aimed at breaking down barriers to competition within and between the public and private sectors, including electricity, gas, and road transport. As noted earlier, the Commonwealth undertook to maintain the pool of FAGs in real per capita terms on a three-year rolling basis, and to make a series of National Competition Payments to the states and territories. The Commonwealth agreed to pay three tranches of the payments commencing in 1997–98 and continuing to 2001–02, depending on states meeting deadlines outlined in the Competition Policy Intergovernmental Agreement and the implementation of specified COAG agreements.

Commenting on the success of COAG, Weller observes that heads of government can take a national view that may make it marginally easier to deal with sectional groups and arguments.[37] As a separate forum from Premiers' Conferences which centre on funding allocations, COAG has the capacity to facilitate discussions aimed at national coordination and jointly negotiated solutions, rather than separate and competing states' interests. In addition to this broad role COAG has dealt with a wide range of issues including microeconomic reforms, social policy (including health and community services), environmental issues, intergovernmental administrative issues, and regulatory reform issues. Its effectiveness in implementing intergovernmental reform on an unprecedented scale is attributed to the commitment of Labor prime ministers (Hawke and Keating) and senior ministers within their governments to the reform agenda, and to the strategic placement of COAG's secretariat within the office of the Prime Minister (PMO) and Cabinet.

From the states' perspective, COAG is seen as a potential "circuit breaker" on Commonwealth centralization of governmental processes and an ongoing forum separate from traditional Premiers' Conferences.[38] Admittedly, COAG's success might be perceived as uneven. It has emphasized microeconomic reform; but it has had less success in negotiations on reforming community services, child care, public housing, the environment, and Native Title, and has not addressed the fundamental reform issue of Commonwealth/ state financial arrangements.[39] Moreover, it has been seen as a Labor invention and has met only three times between 1996 when the Howard government came to office and May 1999. Nevertheless, COAG reforms in program areas have emphasized the shift to output-based funding systems and broadbanded funding of related programs. This has given the states somewhat greater freedom in how they deploy funds, even if it has tightened up requirements that states demonstrate that they are maintaining their own contributions.

In 1995, COAG agreed on the need for major long-term reforms of health and community services. This approach represented a sharing rather than a separation of responsibilities. It sought to have joint setting of Commonweatlh/ state objectives, priorities, performance standards and funding arrangements. The Commonwealth was to take a leadership role in public health standards and research, and the states were to have responsibility for managing and co-ordinating provision of services and for maintaining direct relationships with providers (COAG Communiqué, April 1996). The boundaries of programs were redrawn and grouped into three streams: general care, including community and preventative health and welfare services; acute care; and coordinated care, including a range of specialized services for the frail aged. The aim was to make the individual's needs more important as the basis for planning and funding, to create a funding mechanism that supports better outcomes, to facilitate better linkages between services, and to shift the focus toward total health and community care needs.[40] The reforms incorporated program assignment to a care stream, output-based funding and the model of "care managers"who purchase a mix of services within a set budget. In principle, the agreement marked an important shift of all health and related community services under one multilateral agreement, with bilateral agreements covering funding and outcome measures.

In addition, reforms aimed for improved outcomes for health-care consumers through a variety of provisions: the provision of better information, the coordination of services, a stronger focus on outcomes, investment in prevention and early intervention, moving the planning and management of services as close as possible to the delivery level, and the introduction of incentives for best practices. COAG played an important role in the review of Commonwealth/state responsibilities, the devolution of much service delivery to the states (including the Aged and Community Care Program), and the "broadbanding" of Specific Purpose Payments in public health and health services areas.

The application of National Competition Policy to the health industry has led to the shift to "managed competition" in health. Most important has been the adoption of Casemix as a basis for hospital funding, an innovation that was part of a nationally-initiated attempt at broader reform of hospital management. Casemix is appealing to governments and administrators, but its introduction has been controversial. Length of stay as a funding tool is problematic, and concerns have been raised regarding discharge planning and significant increases in re-admissions following shorter hospital stays.[41] Critics, particularly from the consumer sector and increasingly from doctors and nurses, argue that output-based funding and savings-driven managerialist reforms have undercut the quality of hospital-based health care. There are also arguments that early discharge has shifted costs that were formerly borne by hospitals onto community services and families. With shorter hospital stays, state governments are having to confront increased responsibility for discharge planning and patient care in the community, as well as a need for a mix of high-tech centralized hospitals and other institutions capable of more routine day procedures.

In summary, central to COAG's effectiveness, especially when it met more frequently under Labor up to 1996, has been its location within PMO and

Cabinet, the commitment to a national reform agenda and its involvement of heads of government and senior ministers on agenda items in the national interest. In health, the re-drawing of boundaries into acute care, coordinated care, and general (community and preventative care) has re-set the basis for major funding agreements and outcome measures.

ASSESSING THE EFFECTIVENESS OF INTERGOVERNMENTAL REFORMS

Duckett encapsulates the problems inherent in the intergovernmental system from the point of view of both Commonwealth and state governments. "The different responsibilities of the different players means that the players have different perceptions of the problems of Commonwealth/State relations. Reaching agreement on what the key problems are is thus difficult, making reaching agreement on solutions to those problems even more difficult."[42] From the Commonwealth's point of view, key problems are the escalation of government expenditure on health care, service duplication, and cost-shifting between levels of government, and the difficulty of implementing national priorities. From the states' point of view, the list includes vertical fiscal imbalance and their heavy dependence on Commonwealth funding, Commonwealth-state program overlap, and the conditions attached to tied grants which undermine their autonomy and local diversity in implementation models. To gain a better understanding of these tensions, this section discusses four key issues: rising health-care costs; shifts in the private/public mix of health care; controversies over "tied" grants; and duplication and cost-shifting between levels of government.

Rising Health-Care Costs

Health-care costs, along with quality of care, are major political, social, and economic issues. Rising health-care costs reflect a combination of factors: growth in service intensity and demand pressures, an aging population, growth in biotechnology, system inefficiencies reflecting overlap and duplication of services, inefficient management, cost-shifting from the states to the Commonwealth in areas such as hospital outpatient and emergency services and mental health, a provider-driven medical services system and growth in pharmaceutical expenditures.

In comparison with other Organisation for Economic Co-operation and Development (OECD) countries, Australia been reasonably successful in providing quality health care at a reasonable level of public expenditure. Health expenditure in Australia as a proportion of gross domestic product (GDP) rose from 7.5 percent in 1989–90 to 8.4 percent in 1997–98.[43] This compares with lower expenditures on health in New Zealand and the United Kingdom and higher expenditures in the United States and Canada. However, the cost of health care is growing at a faster rate than the economy as a whole: during the same period, the average annual real growth rate in health expenditure was 4.1 percent, compared to an average annual rate of GDP growth of 3.1 percent. More worrying is the fact that the average rate of health services expenditure growth conceals an uneven distribution over this period; between 1996–97 and 1998–99, the real growth rate of spending on Australian health services increased to 5.1 percent.[44]

Not surprisingly, rising health costs are becoming an intergovernmental issue. Notably, costs have grown more slowly in areas of state responsibility. Compared to the average annual growth rate in Australian recurrent health services expenditure of 4 percent between 1989–90 to 1996–97, expenditure in areas of state responsibility has grown at an annual rate of 3.2 percent for public hospitals, 2.8 percent for nursing homes, and 1.5 percent for ambulance services, and has declined by 5.9 percent in public psychiatric hospitals due to deinstitutionalization. The higher average annual rate of increase in areas of Commonwealth responsibility is especially notable in medical services (4.9 percent) and pharmaceutical services (8.4 percent).[45] Increases in both medical and pharmaceutical services are driven by providers as well as consumers and, as shown in Table 4, these services constitute the two next largest areas of recurrent health expenditure after hospitals.

Federal government budget papers suggest that growth in Commonwealth outlays in health reflect higher utilization of medical and pharmaceutical services with a "drift towards more costly drugs and medical services."[46] Medical services (33.2 percent) and pharmaceutical benefits (13.2 percent) constitute almost half of Commonwealth outlays on health.[47] They thus comprise an interrelated area where outlays are increasing and are difficult to cap. Nevertheless, the government has adopted a number of initiatives, including both demand-side measures such as revoking eligibility for Medicare for some classes of temporary residents, and a variety of supply-side measures such as caps on pathology spending, restrictions on the number of overseas-trained doctors

TABLE 4

Proportion of Recurrent Health Services Expenditure, Current Prices, by Area of Expenditure, 1989–90 to 1996–97 (%)

Area of expenditure	1989–90	1990–91	1991–92	1992–93	1993–94	1994–95	1995–96	1996–97
Total hospitals	40.6	40.1	39.7	38.6	37.7	37.6	37.4	38.1
Public non-psychiatric hospitals	32.3	31.3	30.7	29.8	28.8	28.5	28.2	28.8
Recognized public hospitals	30.6	29.6	29.1	28.2	27.8	27.8	28.2	28.8
Repatriation hospitals	1.7	1.7	1.7	1.5	1.0	0.6	–	–
Private hospitals	6.3	6.9	7.2	7.3	7.5	7.8	8.0	8.4
Private psychiatric hospitals	2.0	1.9	1.8	1.6	1.4	1.3	1.1	0.8
Nursing homes	8.3	8.6	8.4	8.1	7.8	7.5	7.5	7.6
Ambulance	1.5	1.4	1.4	1.4	1.4	1.2	1.3	1.2
Other institutional (necessary)	0.2	0.2	0.2	0.2	0.3	0.3	0.4	–
Total institutional	50.5	50.3	49.8	48.3	47.2	46.6	46.5	46.9
Medical services	18.4	18.7	19.0	19.6	20.0	20.2	19.9	19.7
Other professional services	3.7	3.9	37.0	3.7	3.6	3.6	3.4	3.4
Total pharmaceuticals	9.3	9.5	9.9	10.4	11.0	11.6	11.8	12.2
Benefit paid pharmaceuticals	5.4	5.0	5.2	6.0	6.6	7.0	7.6	7.9
All other pharmaceutical services	3.9	4.5	4.7	4.5	4.4	4.6	4.2	4.3
Aids and appliances	2.1	2.2	2.2	2.2	2.2	2.1	2.0	2.0
Other non-institutional services	14.4	13.8	13.8	14.4	14.4	14.3	14.7	14.2
Community and public health	5.6	4.7	4.4	4.9	5.2	4.7	5.4	5.0
Dental services	5.1	5.3	5.3	5.9	6.0	5.9	6.0	6.1
Administration	3.7	3.8	4.1	3.6	3.2	3.6	3.3	3.1
Research	1.5	1.5	1.5	1.5	1.6	1.6	1.6	1.6
Total non-institutional	49.5	49.7	50.2	51.7	52.8	53.4	53.5	53.1
Total recurrent expenditure	100.0	100.0	100.0	100.0	100.0	100.0	100.0	100.0

Source: AIHW health expenditure database. (AIHW, *Health Expenditure Bulletin No. 15*, p. 16).

entering the medical workforce, and reduced "moonlighting" by temporary resident doctors. Recognizing that much of the problem of unconstrained expenditure centres on private medical practice, attempts have been made to reform primary care. These include: General Practice Grants for activities that are not fee-for-service such as research, evaluation, special training, computer networking; the creation of Divisions of General Practice to work in cooperation with the staff of an area hospital; and piloting the concept of General Practitioners as budget-holders for patients, for example, in the Coordinated Care Trials. As Tables 5 and 6 suggest, trend data provide some evidence that the rate of growth in health-care costs may be slowing, although firm conclusions depend on the area of health expenditure.

Federal-state relations clearly complicate efforts to come to terms with cost pressures. Responsibility for rising health-care costs are consistently "handballed" between Commonwealth and state governments. As Duckett remarks: "there are real problems of Commonwealth/State relations in terms of political process and accountability. The dissipation of responsibility in the health sector means that whenever State or Commonwealth politicians are under pressure they almost inevitably attempt to shift blame to politicians at the other level (the so-called "blame game")."[48]

Shifts in the Private/Public Mix

Shifts in the private/public mix have implications for different levels of government and for total health expenditure, as well as implications for equity and access to services. Two interrelated trends are discussed here: the higher rate of growth of the private hospital system; and recent government policy to encourage the growth of private health insurance. Historically, there has been a mix of private and public providers of hospital care in Australia, with private hospitals mainly run by the non-profit religious sector. Overall, about three-quarters of hospitals are funded from government sources and one-quarter from the private sector. However, this mix is shifting with significant growth in the private hospital sector, the privatization of some public hospitals, and the co-location of private hospitals alongside existing public hospitals. The number of beds in the public system declined by 7,375 between 1993–94 and 1998–99 and the number of private patients being treated in public hospitals has also declined. While funding to public non-psychiatric hospitals as a whole fell from 32.3 to 28.8 percent of recurrent health expenditure between 1989–90 and 1996–97, expenditure on private hospitals rose from 6.3 to 8.4 percent.

TABLE 5
Total Health Services Expenditure, Constant Prices,[a] and Annual Growth Rates, by Source of Funds, 1989–90 to 1997–98

| | Government Sector | | | | Non-government Sector Total[b] | | All Sectors Total | |
| | Commonwealth[b] | | State and Local | | | | | |
Year	Amount	Rate of Growth	Amount	Rate of Growth	Amount	Rate of Growth	Amount	Rate of Growth
1989–90	14,209	2.7	8,670	2.8	10,876	6.6	33,751	3.9
1990–91	14,482	1.9	8,720	0.6	11,323	4.1	34,524	2.3
1991–92	15,140	4.5	8,698	-0.2	11,675	3.1	35,513	2.9
1992–93	16,171	6.8	8,681	-0.2	12,225	4.7	37,077	4.4
1993–94	17,473	8.1	8,259	-4.9	12,862	5.2	38,593	4.1
1994–95	18,127	3.7	8,758	6.1	13,392	4.1	40,278	4.4
1995–96	19,340	6.7	9,387	7.2	13,694	2.3	42,421	5.3
1996–97	19,818	2.5	9,959	6.1	14,503	5.9	44,279	4.4
1997–98[c]	21,199	7.0	10,967	10.1	14,378	-0.1	46,544	5.1
Average annual growth rates[d]								
1989–90 to 1992–93		4.0		0.7		4.6		3.4
1992–93 to 1997–98		5.6		4.8		3.3		4.7
1989–90 to 1997–98		4.9		3.0		3.9		4.1

Notes: [a]Constant price health services expenditure for 1989–90 to 1997–98 is expressed in chain volume measures, reference to the year 1996–97 (see Table 17 of source for major conversion factors used).
[b]Commonwealth government and non-government sector expenditure has been adjusted for tax expenditures. Tax expenditures at constant prices are calculated using chain volume measures with the reference year of 1996–97. The constant price estimates of tax expenditure were: 1989–90 $73 million; 1990–91 $95 million; 1991–92 $89 million; 1992–93 $97 million; 1993–94 $100 million; 1994–95 $95 million; 1995–96 $143 million; 1996–97 $137 million; 1997–98 $179 million in general tax health rebates and $164 million in PHIS tax rebates.
[c]Based on preliminary AIHW and ABS estimates.
[d]Periods covered by these average annual growth rates relate to periods of the Commonwealth/state Medicare agreements.

Source: AIHW health expenditure database (AIHW, *Health Expenditure Bulletin No. 15*, p. 5).

TABLE 6
Capital Expenditure, Constant Prices^a and Annual Growth Rates, by Source of Funds, 1989–90 to 1997–98

Year	Commonwealth		Government Sector State and Local		Total		Non-government Sector		All Sectors	
	Amount ($m)	Rate of Growth (%)	Amount ($m)	Rate of Growth (%)	Amount ($m)	Rate of Growth (%)	Amount ($m)	Rate of Growth (%)	Amount ($m)	Rate of Growth (%)
1989–90	124	..	748	..	872	..	643	..	1506	..
1990–91	164	32.2	806	7.8	970	11.3	499	−21.3	1496	−2.4
1991–92	171	4.3	732	−9.2	902	−7	525	5.2	1427	−2.8
1992–93	138	−19.1	824	12.6	962	6.6	688	31.1	1650	15.6
1993–94	96	−30.6	914	10.9	1009	4.9	843	22.5	1852	12.3
1994–95	8	−91.3	1011	10.7	1020	1.0	802	−4.9	1821	−1.7
1995–96	77	832.5	893	11.7	971	−4.8	818	2.1	1789	−1.8
1996–97	58	−25.2	1122	25.6	1180	21.5	972	18.8	2152	20.3
1997–98^b	64	10.9	1380	23.0	1444	22.4	980	0.7	2424	12.6
Average annual growth rates										
1989–90 to 1992–93		3.7		3.3		3.4		2.8		3.1
1992–93 to 1997–98		−14.2		10.9		8.5		7.3		8.0
1989–90 to 1997–98		−9.1		5.2		3.9		5.5		4.6

Notes: ^aHealth services expenditure for 1989–90 to 1997–98 is expressed in chain volume measures, referenced to 1996–97 using specific health deflators (see Table 17 of source for major deflators used).
^bBased on preliminary AIH and ABS estimates.

Source: AIHW health expenditure database (AIHW, *Expenditure Bulletin No. 15*, p. 18).

Public non-psychiatric hospitals grew at an average annual rate of 2.4 percent over this time compared with 8.4 percent for private hospitals.[49]

As long as a public health system dominates, government can attain a degree of control over expenditure by various means. It does this more successfully with public institutional care, by capping public hospital funding, but it also tries to control expenditures for medical services by setting rebate levels and introducing the reforms to medical practices discussed earlier. Such steps have had a degree of success in curbing expenditure, as evidenced by the modest 0.2 percent growth in health services expenditure between 1996–97 and 1997–98. However, the mix of funding has been changing. The proportion of total health expenditure funded by government fell from 71.9 percent in 1984–85 to 69.1 percent in 1997–98, while non-government expenditure increased from 28.1 percent to 30.9 percent.[50] Private hospitals represent an area where higher costs are met by user payments and private health insurance, and they may therefore be attractive to states as a means of reducing demand for public hospital services for which states are responsible. Looking to the future, growth in private hospitals has the potential to increase overall health-care costs as a proportion of GDP, even if costs to government are unaffected. Such growth could result in a two-tiered health system where more cost-efficient cases are skimmed off by private hospitals, leaving the public system with the higher-cost, longer-stay cases that the private sector is unwilling to treat. Such shifts also impact on retention of skilled medical practitioners and quality of teaching functions in the public system.

Prior to the introduction of Medicare in 1984, up to 78 percent of the population was enrolled in private health insurance.[51] With the introduction of Medicare, coverage had declined to around 30 percent by 1999.[52] Despite this decline, the usage of private hospitals has steadily risen since 1984 and the private hospital sector has grown faster than the public sector in terms of bed days and total admissions,[53] with private health insurers contributing around 70 percent of private hospital expenditure.[54] According to Livingston's analysis, the cost of private health insurance premiums increased by 75 percent from 1989–90 to 1995–96. In comparison, the consumer price index (CPI) increased only 19 percent over the same period. A 1997 Industry Commission inquiry into private health insurance attributed rising premiums to the rise in the proportion of fund members using private rather than public hospitals, rising average private hospital admission charges, increased admissions by private patients, and adverse selection.[55]

Consumer concerns about out-of-pocket fees not covered by private insurance and rising premiums contributed to the dramatic decrease in private insurance membership. With the drop in privately insured patients, pressure on public hospitals has mounted and current government efforts have been directed at increasing private health insurance membership. In 1996, the federal government provided incentives for those privately insured to retain their membership and imposed a financial penalty on high-income earners without such coverage. Then in 1998, the Howard government tax package promised a 30 percent tax rebate to private health policy-holders; and in 1999, it announced the Lifetime Health Cover Scheme, which provides incentives for younger, lower-cost members to take up private health insurance and penalties for older entrants. This measure placed age-related penalties of 2 percent per year on those over 30 who entered after 15 July 2000. Should membership in private health insurance schemes increase markedly, there is concern that shifts to private hospital care could blow out overall health costs and, added to moves by some states to encourage the entry of for-profit providers in privatized public hospitals, radically alter the private-public balance.

This complicated mix of reforms is seen as having the potential to undermine the basic principles of universal access to quality hospital care, a foundation stone of Commonwealth policy. It is not surprising therefore that there is continuing controversy about the commitment of Commonwealth policy to propping up the private health insurance industry with a rebate costing more that $2 billion per year and recorded profits of $126 million by the health insurance companies which had recorded losses in the previous three years.[56] At the time of writing, these measures have had some success in increasing private insurance membership, from 30.5 percent of the Australian population in June 1999 to around 45 percent in mid-2001.[57] However, critics argue that subsidies to the rich in the form of tax rebates for private health insurance could be better used as direct funding to the public hospital and health system. As Owens notes, tensions within the system between Medicare and private health insurance, between stakeholders (medical practitioners, insurers, and private and public hospitals) and between Commonwealth and state governments over cost-shifting, really call for more fundamental review of the whole health system.[58]

Controversies over "Tied" Grants

States have consistently complained that the Commonwealth has forced them to fund its priorities through provisions that require state matching on a dollar-for-dollar basis or through maintenance of effort provisions. States also argue that the detailed reporting requirements of SPPs impose unnecessary administrative costs on the states, and encourage the maintenance of unwieldy and top-heavy Commonwealth bureaucracy. States have drawn on the principle of subsidiarity — locating responsibility for services at the point closest to service delivery — in arguing that they should have primary responsibility for hospital and community services. In this scenario, the Commonwealth would have a role in national benchmark-setting for service delivery in conjunction with the states as service deliverers. States maintain that a shift in responsibilities must be accompanied by measures that "address the States' long term capacity to fund anticipated growth in service demand."[59] An alternative proposal is that in national policy areas such as health, the Commonwealth should bypass the states by directly funding service providers such as hospitals, on the grounds that this would be more efficient and would take away the state's capacity to underspend on health, as illustrated by the use of Medicare funds by Victoria to retire the debt rather than increase hospital spending.

Accountability of states under SPPs is also open to question. In a report on the first attempt to compile a register of SPPs, significant discrepancies were found in the figures provided in the Commonwealth budget and by the Victorian government. This has obvious relevance to assessments of both state and Commonwealth accountability under shared funding agreements and tied grants. The report concluded that such discrepancies are obstacles to achieving a thorough understanding of the impact of SPPs on state government finances.[60]

It is significant that states effectively determine overall levels of service provided in the areas targeted by SPPs and that they can substitute some of the Commonwealth SPP funds for their own contributions,[61] thus freeing their funds for other expenditures such as deficit reduction. This contributes to significant per capita variations in spending between the states in controversial areas of social policy.[62] Such practices have been cited to rebut states' claims for increased health-care payments, with the Commonwealth arguing that states' use of their spending discretion, not Commonwealth limits on funding, have resulted in a "crisis in health." In an audit of SPPs in 1994, the Commonwealth Auditor General questioned program accountability and financial arrangements and identified deficiencies in parliamentary reporting on such grants. Trebeck and Cutbush pinpoint the main problem of SPPs: duplication and overlap have "no offsetting policy coordination or spillover internalising or uniformity of standard benefit for Australia." They argue vertical fiscal imbalance is only partly responsible, and emphasize "deep seated confusion at both levels about the proper role of Government in society in the first place."[63]

Duplication and Cost-shifting between Levels of Government

The report to the Commonwealth Government of the National Commission of Audit (1996) expressed its concerns about the involvement of multiple levels of government. The commission identified cost-shifting as a major problem which would remain even if problems of duplication and overlap were addressed. In the health area, the commission noted that, in response to capped funding and budget constraints in some areas, states have encouraged consumers of health services to switch into uncapped federally-funded programs such as the Medical and Pharmaceutical Benefits Schemes, thereby shifting costs to the Commonwealth. The commission acknowledged that it may be impractical to cede responsibility entirely to one level of government. Even with clear purchaser-provider delineation (e.g., with Commonwealth programs run by the states), it would be difficult to avoid pressures for state involvement in standard-setting or requests for additional funding; and it would also be difficult to avoid Commonwealth involvement in program delivery as a way of verifying costs. The commission concluded that there is no easy solution to this problem, but argued that where practicable, it is best to avoid multiple levels of government involvement in the first place. It therefore pressed for a review of all programs involving multiple levels of government.[64]

The commission argued that the allocation of related programs over different levels of government is a design defect that not only facilitates cost-shifting, but actually creates incentives to engage in such practices. Accordingly, it put forth some program design principles for reducing cost-shifting.[65]

- For programs entirely the responsibility of the states, funding should be in the form of General Purpose Grants, allowing the states allocative discretion between specific programs.
- For programs where there is joint Commonwealth/ state responsibility, funding should go to pools that extend to all related programs, rather than being earmarked to specific programs. Again this would allow the states some allocative discretion within funding pools.
- Where SPPs are considered necessary, the Commonwealth should focus on specifying policy objectives and establishing improved accountability frameworks, and then give the states greater freedom in deciding program delivery. This would facilitate a reduction in the number of SPPs by grouping together or "broadbanding" SPPs which are directed at broad outcomes for particular groups, and would reduce administrative duplication, overlap and inefficiency.[66]

The commission further recommended that the administrative component of retained SPPs should be reduced and argued that any national policy bodies that are retained should be limited to national coordination; strategic directions, and the development of standards, benchmarks, and performance measurements. It took the strong view that the Commonwealth should not be involved in service delivery or approval of projects. These principles have been an important influence on the most recent funding arrangements entered into by the Howard government, in particular the Australian Health Care Agreements and the Public Health Care Agreements. However, it should be borne in mind that not everyone agrees with these policy directions. Critics such as Painter regard "neat and tidy" attempts to sort out clear and distinct roles and responsibilities as misreading the constitutional logic of Australian federalism. "It ignores the essential feature of concurrence in the division of powers in the Australian Constitution, and the adversarial and competitive dynamic of Australian federal politics."[67]

CONCLUSION

The Commonwealth's dominance over the financial operation of the federation in Australia has arisen largely because of the High Court's interpretation of the Constitution which has allowed the Commonwealth government's wartime monopoly over income taxation to continue. As a result, the most notable aspect of Australian Commonwealth-state relations is extreme vertical fiscal imbalance, marked by the Commonwealth's control of major tax bases and the states' responsibility for most expenditure and service provisions. Tax reform is one attempt to address this issue, although it is too early to judge its effectiveness.

The provision of SPPs or "tied" grants to the states under section 96 of the Constitution has enabled the Commonwealth to expand its role in the health system. Controversy surrounding tied grants is ongoing. From the Commonwealth perspective, SPPs satisfy demands for minimum national standards in areas such as health, with the Commonwealth setting strategic goals and fostering states' optional provision of services from available resources. From their point of view, the states prefer fewer restrictions and view matched funding arrangements as restricting their budgetary flexibility, especially where such arrangements have not been agreed to on a cooperative basis. States perceive this as the Commonwealth government dictating the terms of service provision and advancing its own interests. They also argue that SPPs result in unnecessary state/Commonwealth duplication and overlap, and reduce state government flexibility and responsiveness. States have been vocal in their continued complaints of funding shortfalls which inhibit their capacity to deliver services to taxpayers.

Much of the body of this chapter has focused on unravelling Commonwealth/state funding of health and the role of institutions, such as COAG, in forging a more effective and efficient national agenda in health. This agenda demands a national system with the capacity to generate comprehensive national policies related to health care and to implement national microeconomic reforms. It also demands that the system adequately balance efficiency with equity and quality of care issues, that intergovernmental institutions facilitate better and more efficient Commonwealth government/state cooperation, and that the system address unmet needs, especially in aged and disability care. Ongoing difficulties in policy implementation rely on negotiations with the states and give rise to distortions of priorities or goal-shifting in the implementation phase. These issues really frame the challenge of effective intergovernmental relations.

Broadbanded and outcome-based Commonwealth funding is an increasing trend. This entails the bracketing of SPPs, where funds are provided for broad outcomes rather than for more specific activities, and states make decisions in line with National Competition Policy on how to employ funds to meet designated Commonwealth objectives. This might satisfy their desire for more choice as to how they deploy funds but, as some critics observe, it could lead to the decline of uniformity and poor achievement of national goals and national oversight of some specific programs (such as women's health) submerged within broadbanded pooling of funds. Many of these reforms are, as Duckett notes, located at the margins. He proposes a more radical but politically unlikely possiblility that all responsibility for health and community services could be assigned to one level of government.

The health issues that dominate the policy agenda in Australia are similar to those in many other countries, federal and non-federal alike: cost containment, demographic pressures, the implications of changing medical technologies, shifting balances among stakeholders, and increasingly neo-liberal policy orientations to government generally. Moreover, federalism does not prevent a broadly national response to this daunting policy agenda. The Commonwealth plays a central role in policy-setting, directly establishing critical parameters for health insurance programs and providing leadership in the joint development of influential national policies and standards in forums such as COAG. Nevertheless, federalism does inject another set of issues into the politics of health care, issues specific to the management of a complex system of intergovernmental interdependence: a continuing tension between cohesive national policies and local discretion and flexibility; concerns about accountability of governments for the expenditure of public funds; problems of cost-shifting, and other inefficiencies inherent in a complex system of fiscal arrangements. None of these tensions are new. But in an era increasingly focused on the efficient delivery of services to the public, the complexities and incentives embedded in intergovernmentalism pose more obvious problems. Clearly, the classic tensions between national politics and federal institutions remain as vibrant as ever in Australia.

NOTES

I am grateful to Josephine Muir and Sally Cowling for assistance with gathering information for this research.

[1]Australian doctors divide into two main practice groups: specialists and general practitioners (GPs) who deliver primary health-care services as the first point of entry to medical treatment. Under Medicare, GPs have the choice of bulk-billing some or all patients. This means the government will automatically reimburse 85 percent of the schedule fee for the consultation. Health Care Card holders (qualifying Department of Social Security pension and benefit recipients) are bulk-billed as an equity measure under Medicare. For non-Health Care Card holders, GPs may bill the patient for the full cost of a consultation, leaving it to the patient to recoup the 85 percent reimbursement. Specialist fees which are only part-reimbursed under Medicare, involve a higher proportion of user contribution to the cost of consultations. See S. Hill, "Consumer Payments for Health Care," in *Health Policy in the Market State*, ed. L. Hancock (St. Leonards: Allen & Unwin, 1999), for an analysis of health-care consumers' out-of-pocket expenses.

[2]As defined by the Australian Institute of Health and Welfare (AIHW), *Australia's Health 1998* (Canberra: Australian Government Publishing Service, 1998), p. 164.

[3]While much of the debate on funding focuses on government expenditure, it should also be acknowledged that a growing proportion of Australians seek out alternative therapists; estimated at over $1 billion spent on alternative medicines and therapists. See G.P. Atkin and S. Kristoffersen, "Alternative Medicine: An Expanding Health Industry," *Medical Journal of Australia* 166 (May 1997):516; and K. Bisset, "Alternative Medicine: Patients Spend $1b," *Australian Doctor*, 8 March 1996, p. 1. A growing number of doctors are practising alternative medicine, and some are charging up-front fees. However, more research is needed to factor private expenditures on alternative therapies into discussions of health-care spending.

[4]The Australian Commonwealth comprises six states (Victoria, New South Wales, Queensland, Western Australia, South Australia, Tasmania) and two territories, the Northern Territory and the Australian Capital Territory. In subsequent discussion reference to states will be taken to include territories.

[5]Local government has no formal recognition in the Commonwealth Constitution. However, since 1996 the Council of Australian Governments has recognized the significant role played by local government in areas of health and community services. Local government typically encompasses cities, towns, shires, boroughs, municipalities, and district councils; with a focus on road and bridge construction and maintenance, water sewerage and drainage systems, health and sanitation services, building supervision and administration of regulations; along with some service provision in recreation, culture, and community services. Its revenue source comprises direct grants from the Commonwealth (about 20 percent of revenue). State government grants and local government revenue — mainly property rates along with fines and service charges.

[6]H. Emy and O. Hughes, *Australian Politics: Realities in Conflict*, 2d ed. (Melbourne: Macmillan, 1991), p. 305.

[7]Federal-State Relations Committee, *Australian Federalism: The Role of the States*, Second Report of the Inquiry into Overlap and Duplication (Melbourne: Government Printer, 1998), p. xvii. For a summary of the background to federation in its earlier years, see J. Summers, "Federalism and Commonwealth-State Relations," in *Government, Politics, Power and Policy in Australia*, ed. A. Parkin, J. Summers and D. Woodward, 5th ed. (Melbourne: Longman-Cheshire); and regarding later periods, see C. Fletcher, "Responsive Government: Duplication and Overlap in the Australian Federal System," Discussion Paper No. 3 (Canberra: Federalism Research Centre, 1991).

[8]B. Galligan, "What is the Future of the Federation?" *Journal of Public Administration* 55, 3(1996):78-79.

[9]Federal-State Relations Committee, *Australian Federalism*, p. xx.

[10]The High Court of Australia has powers granted under the Constitution to review Commonwealth and state legislation in terms of its constitutionality. Several state challenges to Commonwealth dominance over uniform income taxation have failed.

[11]Federal-State Relations Committee, *Australian Federalism*, p. xxii.

[12]S. Duckett, "Commonwealth/State Relations in Health," in *Health Policy in the Market State*, ed. Hancock.

[13]Ibid., p. 71.

[14]See Australian Health Ministers, *Second National Mental Health Plan* (Canberra: Commonwealth of Australia, 1998).

[15]Druckett, "Commonwealth/State Relations in Health," p. 71.

[16]The main payments in this category relate to non-governmental schools and local government general purpose assistance. Funds paid "to" the states (a small number of Special Purpose Payments made direct to local government) relate to child-care

programs administered by local governments on behalf of the Commonwealth and funding for aged and disabled persons' homes and hostels. In terms of federal-state funding however, grants to local government constitute only a small proportion of total Commonwealth assistance (4.3 percent) and will not be discussed separately.

[17]Australian Institute of Health and Welfare (AIHW), *Health Expenditure Bulletin No. 15: Australia's Health Services Expenditures to 1997-98* (Canberra: AIHW, 1999), p. 5.

[18]See D. James, *Commonwealth Assistance to the States Since 1976*, Background Paper No. 5 (Canberra: Parliamentary Library, Parliament of Australia, 1997), p. 2; Federal-State Relations Committee, *Report on the Register of Specific Purpose Payments Received by Victoria*, Fourth Report of the Inquiry into Overlap and Duplication, Vols. 1 and 2 (Melbourne: Government Printer, 1999).

[19]Commonwealth of Australia, *1999 Budget Papers* (Canberra: Australian Government Publishing Service, 1999), No. 1 Table 1 and No. 3 Chart 3.

[20]Commonwealth payments to the states and territories may also take the form of payments for recurrent or capital purposes, general purpose capital assistance (such as the Building Better Cities Program, loans to the States [the Loans Council Program was abolished by the Keating government in 1994–95] and National Competition payments, from 1995).

[21]Commonwealth of Australia, *1999 Budget Papers.*

[22]General Revenue Assistance is paid as Financial Assistance Grants, which were put in place in 1942–43 to compensate states for Commonwealth wartime levying of income taxation. The level of grants is indexed to annual movements in the Consumer Price Index and projections of population as at 31 December each year. Indexation is guaranteed on a rolling three-year basis subject to states complying with obligations under the 1995 COAG agreement to implement National Competition Policy and related reforms. Other forms of General Revenue Assistance include: Special Revenue Assistance Grants to the Northern Territory and the Australian Capital Territory (0.07 of general revenue assistance); and National Competition Payments, which are conditional on states' compliance with the obligations of the 1995 Council of Australian Governments Agreement (2.3 percent of general revenue assistance).

[23]Commonwealth of Australia, *1998-99 Budget Paper No. 3* (Canberra: Australian Government Publishing Service, 1998), p. 17.

[24]James, *Commonwealth Assistance to the States*, p. 1.

[25]Commonwealth of Australia, *2001 Budget Paper No. 1 and No. 3* (Canberra: Australian Government Publishing Service, 2001).

[26]With implementation of the intergovernmental agreement on the reform of Commonwealth-State Financial Relations from 1 July 2000 (with the introduction of the goods and services tax), general assistance to local government will become the responsibility of the states and the Northern Territory (Commonwealth of Australia, *1999 Budget Paper No. 3*, ch. 3, p. 16).

[27]AIHW, *Health Expenditure Bulletin No. 5*, p. 6.

²⁸James, *Commonwealth Assistance to the States*, pp. 15-29; Commonwealth of Australia, *1999 Budget Paper No. 3*, ch. 3, p. 17 and *2001 Budget Paper No. 3*, p. 5.

²⁹Under the agreement attached to *A New Tax System* (Commonwealth-State Financial Arrangements) *Act 1999*, the following provisions apply. *Budget Paper No. 3*, pp. 108-24:

1. Payment of FAGs (Financial Assistance Grants) to states will cease on 1 July 2000;
2. The Commonwealth will continue to pay SPPs to the states and has no intention of cutting aggregate SPPs as part of this reform process;
3. Transitional arrangements to assist the states will include interest-free loans July 2000–01;
4. Any proposal to vary the 10 percent rate will need unanimous support of all states and territory governments and Commonwealth government endorsement with passage by both houses of Parliament;
5. A ministerial council comprising Commonwealth and state treasurers will oversee the implementation of the agreement and consider ongoing reform of Commonwealth-state financial relations;
6. The Commonwealth will distribute GST revenue grants among the states and territories in accordance with horizontal fiscal equalization principles and the pool of funding will comprise GST revenue grants and health-care grants (as defined under the Australian Health Care Agreement);
7. A state's share of the pool will be based on population share and a relativity factor based on Commonwealth Grants Commission recommendations.

³⁰See C. Walsh, "Federal Reform and the Politics of Vertical Fiscal Imbalance," *Australian Journal of Political Science* 27 (Special Issue, 1992):19-38; James, *Commonwealth Assistance to the States*; Federal-State Relations Committee, *Report on the Register of Specific Purpose Payments*, Vol. 2.

³¹Australia has a bicameral system of government with upper and lower houses. Framers of the Australian Constitution saw the Senate as a means of protecting state/ territory from being dominated by political party influences. But as argued by numerous commentators, in reality, the Senate does not function as a states/territories' house. See J. Warden, "Federalism and the Design of the Australian Constitution," Discussion Paper No. 19 (Canberra: Federalism Research Centre, 1992).

³²Hawke's New Federalism is important for its commitment to responsiveness to local needs and the needs of regional diversity, delivery of quality cost-effective services (removing duplication between various government levels), a competitive national economy based on "competitive federalism," a guaranteed revenue base that matches states' and territories' expenditure responsibilities and a federation that is accountable through Parliament (Leader's Forum, 1994). Four principles mark Labor Prime Minister Hawke's New Federalism: the Australian Nation principle; the subsidiary principle; the structural efficiency principle and the accountability principle (K. Wiltshire, "The Directions of Constitutional Change: Implications for the Public

Sector," *Australian Journal of Public Administration* 55(3):90-96, p. 94). While these reforms are mainly discussed as cooperative federalism, Painter notes that state government leaders have articulated a model of "competitive federalism" as a way of justifying their autonomy as a defence against Commonwealth domination of collaborative institutions. M. Painter, "After Managerialism: Rediscoveries and Redirections, the Case of Intergovernmental Relations," paper given at Public Policy and Private Management Conference, University of Melbourne, May 1998.

[33]M. Painter, "The Council of Australian Governments and Intergovernmental Relations: A Case of Cooperative Federalism," *Publius* 26 (1996):101.

[34]The Leader's Forum, established in 1994, has been an important adjunct to the involvement of states/territories' in COAG, allowing state leaders to meet to develop a cooperative approach in their dealings with the Commonwealth.

[35]E. Harman and F. Harman, "The Potential for Local Diversity in Implementation of the National Competition Policy," *Australian Journal of Public Administration* 55 (3):12-25.

[36]States and territories agreed with its principles, subject to the proviso that recommendations apply to all Commonwealth- and state government-owned enterprises; and that states and territories share in the benefits of reform and privatization of State Trading Enterprises and have the capacity to authorize exemptions from the *Trade Practices Act.*

[37]P. Weller, "Commonwealth-State Reform Processes: A Policy Management Review," *Australian Journal of Public Administration* 55,1 (1996):104.

[38]P. Hendy, "Intergovernmental Relations," *Australian Journal of Public Administration* 55,1 (1996):111-12.

[39]Ibid., p. 112.

[40]Council of Australian Governments (COAG) Task Force on Health and Community Services, "Health and Community Services: Meeting People's Needs Better," Discussion Paper (Canberra: Australian Government Printing Service, 1995), pp. 11-12.

[41]M. Draper, "Casemix: Financing Hospital Services," in *Health Policy in the Market State*, ed. Hancock.

[42]S. Duckett, "Commonwealth/State Relations in Health," p. 73.

[43]AIHW, *Health Expenditure Bulletin No. 15*, p. 2.

[44]Ibid., p. 3.

[45]Ibid., p. 17.

[46]Commonwealth of Australia, *Budget Strategy and Outlook, 1997-98, Budget Paper No. 1* (Canberra: Australian Government Publishing Service, 1997), pp. 4.41-42.

[47]Australian Institute of Health and Welfare, *Australia's Health 2000* (Canberra: Australian Government Publishing Service, 2000), p. 40.

[48]Drucket, "Commonwealth/State Relations in Health," p. 78.

[49]AIHW, *Health Expenditure Bulletin No. 15*, pp. 16-17; and R. Crowley, *Healing our Hospitals: A Report into Public Hospital Funding* (Canberra: Parliament of Australia, Senate Community Affairs References Committee, 2000), p. 9.

[50]Ibid., pp. 2-5; AIHW, *2000 Budget Papers*, p. 407.

[51]H. Owens,"Health Insurance," in *Economics and Australian Health Policy*, ed. G. Mooney and R. Scotton (St. Leonards: Allen & Unwin, 1998), p. 175.

[52]The areas where private health insurance makes some contribution and consumers contribute substantially to costs are those not covered by Medicare, such as private hospitals, specialist medical fees, dental services, non-medical professional services, aids, and appliances.

[53]C. Livingston, "Private Health Insurance: A Triumph for Market Ideology," *Health Issues* 51 (1997):28.

[54]AIHW, *Australia's Health 1998*, p. 288.

[55]Industry Commission, *Private Health Insurance, Report No. 57* (Canberra: Australian Government Publishing Service, 1997).

[56]Standard and Poors, *Australia Health Insurers Report* (2000). At <www.standardandpoors. com>.

[57]Private Health Insurance Administration Council (PHIAC), *News Bulletin* (Canberra: PHIAC, 1999).

[58]Owens, "Health Insurance," p. 191.

[59]Australian Capital Territory Government, Intergovernmental Financial Relations, *Budget Paper No. 3* (Canberra: ACT Government, 1998), p. 6.

[60]Federal-State Relations Committee, *Report on the Register of Specific Purpose Payments*, p. 39.

[61]D. Moore 1996, "Duplication and Overlap: An Exercise in Federal Power," *Upholding the Australian Constitution*, Proceedings of the 6th Conference of the Samuel Griffith Society, November, pp. 37-64.

[62]A recent study focused on patterns of expenditure in the State of Victoria and drawing on budget data, showed that state spending on education, health, community services, and welfare had fallen from 6.48 to 6.17 percent of gross state product between 1991–92 and 1998–99. Drawing on Commonwealth Grants Commission data the study found that social spending in Victoria (on health, education, and welfare) had fallen 10.7 percent or $281 per head of population over the five years from 1993–94 to 1997–98 and that by 1997–98, Victoria was behind the average of the other Australian states by $138 in education, $174 in health, and $8 in welfare. See L. Hancock and S. Cowling, *Searching for Social Advantage: What Has Happened to the "Social Dividend" for Victorians?* (Carleton: Centre for Public Policy, University of Melbourne, 1999).

[63]D. Trebeck and G. Cutbush, *Overlap and Duplication in Federal-State Relations* (Sydney: Samuel Griffith Society, 1996), p. 8.

[64]It asked that the following questions be addressed: Whether Commonwealth involvement is the only solution, even where national standards of service delivery

are considered desirable; whether uniform standards could be maintained as a result of state level cooperation or competition; whether the states acting together as competitors could deliver acceptable programs and standards, in which case the Commonwealth could vacate the field. See National Commission of Audit, *Report to the Commonwealth/National Commission of Audit* (Canberra: Australian Government Publishing Service, 1996), p. 47.

[65]Ibid., pp. 47-48.

[66]Ibid., p. 48.

[67]Painter, "After Managerialism," p. 8.

5

FEDERAL-STATE RELATIONS IN UNITED STATES HEALTH POLICY

David C. Colby

In the United States, relationships between federal and state governments are constitutionally ambiguous. Divisions of powers are not neat and tidy. Few clear jurisdictional lines exist, even within a single policy arena. The Constitution of 1789, court cases, culture, and practice have influenced the development of federal-state relations in a peculiar way.

Much of intergovernmental relations in health care are based on a grant-in-aid system. States can choose whether to participate in individual grant programs or not. Even after accepting a grant from the federal government, states have much flexibility, allowing for considerable programmatic variation across states within broad federal rules. More flexibility is allowed through the use of waivers to the federal policies. Flexibility does not provide a solution to conflict and comes at a high cost, however. Conflict arises due to differences in views of federal-state relations and the role of the public sector, but, most importantly, due to the cost of programs and the rules for receiving grants. The high degree of policy flexibility allows for inequity in how individuals in the same circumstances are treated across states.

This chapter will cover several topics toward an understanding of US federal-state relations in health care. It begins with a description of federalism, including the constitutional principles, especially as they apply to health care and the grants-in-aid system. This is followed by a description of the US health-care system, and intergovernmental relations in health care, including the Medicaid program, the Children's Health Insurance Program, and regulation of the health-care sector. Finally, there is an assessment of health-care federalism in the United States.

FEDERALISM

This section first presents a description of the constitutional provisions, especially those that affect health policy. It follows with a consideration of grants-in-aid as the major intergovernmental mechanism in the US system.

Constitutional Provisions

In advocating the adoption of the Constitution of 1789, James Madison, writing under the pseudonym Publius, described it as "neither wholly federal not wholly national."[1] Thus, the allocation of powers in the United States is, as Thomas Anton has termed it, "ambiguous."[2] That allocation has varied over time. The principles for allocation of power are based on constitutional provisions: enumerated powers, including the power to tax, the power over interstate commerce, and reserved powers. Enumerated powers are those granted to the national government by the Constitution (article 1, section 8). Most of these are very specific (e.g., the power to establish post offices). The Constitution, however, grants the power to pass laws that are necessary and proper to carry out the enumerated powers of the national government. This provision creates implied powers, providing much legal elasticity for the meager list of enumerated powers in the Constitution. Early in our history, the Supreme Court supported the notion of implied powers.[3]

Not surprisingly, given our eighteenth-century constitution, there is no discussion of power over health care. Two of the enumerated powers, however, are broad and would later influence the development of health policy. One of these is the power to tax and, by implication, spend for the general welfare. In arguing for the adoption of the Constitution, James Madison viewed the general welfare clause as tied directly to enumerated powers.[4] In 1854, President Franklin Pierce vetoed a federal grant-in-aid program for the indigent insane with a similar narrow interpretation of the general welfare clause. Nevertheless, in the twentieth century, especially since the 1930s, the Supreme Court has given a broad interpretation of the general welfare clause.[5] Today, the power to tax and spend for the general welfare is not limited to the enumerated powers of the federal government.

The second important provision is the power to regulate interstate commerce. Surprisingly early in the development of the United States, the issue of interstate commerce arose. In 1798, New York granted a monopoly over steamboat navigation on the waterways in the state. Two issues arose in that situation. First, what was commerce? The Supreme Court decided that commerce included all species of commercial intercourse. Second, what is interstate? The Supreme Court ruled, "Commerce among states cannot stop at the external boundary line of each state, but may be introduced into the interior."[6] Although states could not interfere with interstate commerce, the federal government did not have exclusive power over commerce.[7] There, however, was little affirmative exercise of this power by the federal government until the twentieth century. State legislation was generally upheld when there was no federal legislation or when the commerce affected was clearly local. For example, in 1869 the Supreme Court upheld state regulation of insurance even though it was sold across state lines because it was not commerce.[8] Nevertheless, today the federal government can regulate insurance sold across state lines, but generally has delegated that power to state governments.[9]

All powers not granted to the federal government by the Constitution are reserved to the states or the people (article X). Although this provision is viewed as weak, states clearly retained police powers when they joined the United States.[10] Police powers are those powers that affect health, welfare, and morals. The federal commerce power and state police power could (and have) come into conflict. The Supreme Court has stated that the principal protection for state power when it is in conflict with federal commerce power lies in the political process in which states are key players.[11]

Although the commerce clause and taxing and spending for the general welfare have supported broad federal interventions in social and economic policy, there remain some limits to these powers. For example, a federal law outlawing the possession of a gun in a school zone could not be justified under the commerce clause. The commerce clause can be used to sustain laws that keep interstate commerce "free from immoral and injurious uses"; may protect interstate commerce even though the threat may come from intrastate activities; and be used to regulate those activities that have a substantial relation to interstate commerce.[12] Nevertheless, this case, as John Kincaid noted, "hoists the Tenth Amendment another inch back up the constitutional flagpole."[13] More recent Supreme Court cases had continued this trend in strengthening state power.[14]

The one exception to the ambiguous nature of the United States federal system is the relationship between state and local governments. Localities are not autonomous units, but organizations whose existence depends on state governments. Dillon's rule, espoused in 1868 by an Iowa judge, enunciates the principle that localities are creatures of the state and can exercise only those powers expressly granted by the state. Thus, cities, counties, and other local governmental units have little flexibility in the development of policy. From 1789 to 1860, the United States had a period of dual federalism in which federal and state governments generally exercised power in separate realms. The federal government, nevertheless, provided western states with land for common schools, assumed state revolutionary war debts, and distributed some funds from the sale of national lands and from treasury surpluses to the states.[15]

Between 1861 and 1930, dual federalism began to break down. The development of our national economy raised conflicts between state police power and federal commerce power. Also, in that period, we began to develop federal programs that provided grants of money to states. By 1900 there were five grant programs, providing federal money to state governments. By 1930 there were 15 such programs. Between 1930 and 1960 we had a period of cooperative federalism in which there were shared responsibilities between federal and state governments. From 1960 to about 1980 there was a period of conflict between federal and state governments. Certainly since the Reagan administration (some would argue as early as the Carter administration), there has been more balance in the power relationship between the federal and state governments, and some trend toward decentralization.[16]

Intergovernmental Mechanism

The mechanism that dramatically changed the relationship between the federal and state governments was the use of grants by the federal government to promote social policies. While grants of money and land by the federal government were used in the nineteenth century, they were directed mainly at agriculture and schools.

One of the first grant programs dealing with the health policy was the *Maternity Act* of 1921, which provided funds to states to reduce maternal and infant mortality. Massachusetts challenged its constitutionality on the grounds that "these appropriations are for purposes not federal, but local to the states, and together with numerous similar appropriations constitute an effective means of inducing the states to yield a portion of their sovereign rights."[17] The Supreme

Court, however, ruled that the powers of the state were not infringed "since the act imposed no obligation, but simply extends an option which the state is free to accept or reject."[18] This principle was affirmed later in other policy areas.[19]

In the first year of the *Maternity Act*, 40 states accepted money and by the end of 1927, 45 states had accepted money.[20] Although the Act was not renewed (ending in 1929) because of opposition from the American Medical Association, nativist groups, and others it became the model for intergovernmental health programs. It was a categorical grant program with state financial matching and federal standards.[21]

The *Federal Emergency Relief Act* of 1933 was the first instance of a federal grant program for welfare. This was followed in 1935 by the *Social Security Act* which provided for a national retirement program (commonly referred to as Social Security) as well as grant programs to support state welfare programs for dependent children, and blind and poor elderly individuals. In upholding the *Social Security Act*, the Supreme Court noted that:

> during the years 1929 to 1936, when the country was passing through a cyclical depression, the number of the unemployed mounted to unprecedented heights.... The fact developed quickly that the states were unable to give the requisite relief. The problem had become national in area and dimensions. There was need of help from the nation if the people were not to starve. It is too late today for the argument to be heard with tolerance that in a crisis so extreme that the use of the moneys of the nation to relieve the unemployed and their dependents is a use for any other purpose than promotion of the general welfare.[22]

While most of the *Social Security Act* dealt with income support policies, there were provisions that provided for grants to states for maternal and child health, and for strengthening state and local health departments.

After World War II, Congress passed the Hill-Burton Act, which provided for grants for surveys of hospital needs and for construction of hospitals. This was followed in the 1960s and 1970s by grant programs for state and local health planning. In 1960 Congress passed the Kerr-Mills program, which was a grant program to furnish medical care to low-income elderly persons. That program was seen primarily as a supplement to public assistance and as a means to shift the burden for financing to the federal government.[23] It had joint federal-state financing, state administration in accordance with federal standards, and eligibility tied to state standards for welfare. In 1965 Kerr-Mills was replaced by the Medicaid program, which while broadening coverage used the Kerr-Mills model for intergovernmental relations.

Federal grants to state, local, and non-governmental units take many forms in the United States. They involve different degrees of federal control over their distribution and over the use of funds. Variation in the degree of control over distribution ranges from formula grants which are awarded by a fixed rule to all governmental units that qualify, to project grants, which are awarded for specific undertakings. Variation in the degree of control over the use of funds ranges from block grants that are awarded for broad purposes to categorical grants that are awarded narrower purposes.[24]

HEALTH-CARE SYSTEM

Characterizing the US health-care system is difficult even for an audience in the United States. For example, over half of Americans who are covered by managed-care insurance say that they have never been in managed care.[25] For Canadians and Europeans, gaining an understanding of this system must seem formidable and those who do may see the US system as peculiar.

The US health-care system is undergoing profound changes. It is moving rapidly to a market-based system, emphasizing competition, consumer choice, and personal responsibility. It is pluralistic, even within one sector of the industry. Much of our delivery and insurance systems are merged in managed-care products. With the development of managed care, power is shifting from providers to insurers. The backlash against managed care is partially a fight to regain control. The system is also moving from its non-profit historical roots to a more for-profit basis. Some non-profit institutions are converting to for-profit status, while others are retaining their status, but behaving like for-profit entities. Most importantly, it is not one system, but varies by market and state.[26] To paraphrase the late Congressman Thomas O'Neill's statement about politics, all health care in the United States is local.

Health Policies

Prior to World War II, federal government involvement in health care was directed mainly at merchant marines, Indians, and military veterans.[27] The first involvement was the development of a marine hospital service in 1798. It was not until 1893 that the service was given responsibility over interstate and foreign quarantine. In 1903 the Public Health and *Marine Hospital Service Act* was passed, giving additional authority over the sale of biologic products. In 1906, the *Pure Foods and Drug Act* banned adulterated and mislabelled food and drugs from interstate commerce, giving the public health service some more authority. Much of health policy is an extension of welfare policy. Based on English poor law, welfare was considered a local function until the 1930s.[28] In early Massachusetts, for example, towns were responsible for their poor and the state was responsible for the "unsettled" poor. Later states established financial aid programs for the deserving poor, including the insane, the blind, and the disabled.[29]

Today, the United States has three major health programs. *Medicare*, a health insurance program, which serves nearly 40 million elderly and disabled persons, is a federal program with few direct intergovernmental aspects (except as noted below). *Medicaid*, a health insurance program that was targeted mainly to the welfare poor, is a joint federal-state program; the *State Child Health Insurance Program*, which is a new health insurance program directed at poor children, is also a joint federal-state program.

Health Financing

The United States relies on private and public institutions as well as individuals to finance health care. In general, the explicit public role is limited to helping special, "deserving" populations. But there are hidden ways that the system provides subsidies for others through the tax law.

Health care is financed predominately by private sources, accounting for about 53 percent of expenditures. These private sources include private health insurance (33 percent), out-of-pocket payments paid by individuals (16 percent), and other sources (4 percent).[30] The federal government pays about one-third of expenditures with state and local government contributing about 13 percent of health expenditures.[31]

Health Insurance

Although private health insurance was available in the early 1900s, few Americans had insurance until after World War II. In the economic depression of the 1930s, hospitals introduced insurance to help individuals pay for hospitalization.[32] At that time, the American Medical Association, however, opposed even private insurance to cover physician services.[33] During World War II, the Internal Revenue Service (IRS) ruled that employer contributions to health insurance would not be taxed as income. With a wartime freeze on wages, employers began to offer health insurance as a way to provide additional compensation to employees. In 1953 the IRS reversed its decision. Then in 1954 Congress amended the Internal Revenue Code to exclude the cost of employer-provided health insurance coverage from gross income. That provision remains in force today. Self-employed individuals also can deduct up to 45 percent of the cost of health insurance premiums from taxable income.[34] These and related tax provisions are worth about $266 billion in foregone tax revenues.[35]

For non-elderly persons, employers are the overwhelming source of insurance. In 1996, slightly less than two-thirds of the non-elderly received health insurance from employers. About 15 percent received insurance from public sources with Medicaid being the leading source. Fewer than 7 percent had insurance coverage purchased in the individual market. In the non-elderly group, most people with insurance are in managed-care products that limit to some degree the delivery system choices available to them. In 1997, 30 percent of insured employees were in health maintenance organizations (HMOs). Fifty-five percent were in other types of managed-care products.[36] HMOs are paid capitated monthly fees to provide all needed covered health-care services for the enrolled population. In some managed-care organizations, payments are also capitated to physicians or practices for a subset of the services.

About 18 percent of non-elderly Americans were uninsured. The percentage of uninsured persons has grown in the last decade due to three factors. First, between the late 1980s and now some employers have dropped health insurance.[37] Second, a higher proportion of employees are refusing employer-based coverage, presumably due to unaffortability of coverage;[38] and finally, welfare reform led to decreases in the number of people covered by Medicaid. The Medicare program serves about 40 million beneficiaries. Medicare covers virtually all people over age 65 and about 5 million disabled individuals under age 65. Eighty-two percent of beneficiaries are in traditional Medicare, which is a government administered fee-for-service plan. Others are in private health maintenance organizations. The *Balanced Budget Act* of 1997 created a program called Medicare+Choice, which offers Medicare beneficiaries three options in addition to traditional Medicare. These are coordinated health plans (health maintenance organizations, preferred provided organizations and provider-sponsored organizations), private fee-for-service plans, and on a demonstration basis, medical savings accounts. Among those Medicare beneficiaries in traditional Medicare, about 87 percent have supplemental insurance coverage. Most purchase private supplemental insurance or have employer-provided supplemental insurance. About 15 percent have Medicaid.[39]

Health-Care Delivery System

In the last few years, the health-care providers have been losing power to in-surers. There is also a considerable consolidation and integration occurring in this sector. The delivery system includes about 5,000 general hospitals, 750,000 physicians, and numerous allied health professionals. About one-third of health-care spending is for hospitals and about one-fifth is for physicians. Spending on in-patient hospital services has been decreasing dramatically and hospital occupancy rates are dropping.

At the local level, there are substantial efforts to merge hospitals into systems, alliances or partnerships. In many places, hospitals are also forming partnerships with physician practices. Some non-profit hospitals and public hospitals are switching to for-profit status, allowing them to use equity mar-kets for financing. Finally, physician practices are consolidating. Short-term, acute-care, non-federal hospitals deliver most of the hospital care in the United States. Of the slightly more than 5,000 short-term, acute-care hospitals, non-profit organizations own about 3,000, state and local governments own about 1,200, and for-profit corporations own a small number.[40] Federal hospitals are for military personnel and veterans.

Of the 750,000 physicians, about 82 percent are delivering patient care. Of those delivering care, 35 percent are primary physicians. About three-quarters of physicians have office-based practices and the remainder are in hospital-based practices.[41]

INTERGOVERNMENTAL RELATIONS IN HEALTH CARE

Federal-state relationships in the United States are very program specific. Even within particular policy areas, the intergovernmental relationships differ by program. In this consideration of health policy, I focus on Medicaid, the pro-gram that dominates intergovernmental relations in health policy. Medicaid constitutes over 90 percent of federal intergovernmental health expenditures. Nevertheless, other health programs will be discussed in order to provide some comparisons.

Medicaid

Medicaid is a joint federal-state program providing payment for medical and related services to approximately 36 million low-income persons who are predominately aged, blind, disabled, or members of families with dependent children. It has had three distinct features: joint federal-state financing, state administration in accordance with broad federal standards, and eligibility tied to state standards for other cash benefits. Recently, the link with eligibility for cash benefits has been severed. Although broad federal guidelines determine eligibility and coverage standards, each state designs and administers its own Medicaid program. As a result, state programs vary considerably in eligibility requirements, service coverage, utilization limits, provider payment policies, and use of managed care.

Service Coverage and Limitations

Under the current program, all states must provide a standard benefit package to the categorically needy that includes inpatient and outpatient hospital services; physician services; laboratory and X-ray services; family planning; skilled nursing facility (SNF) services for adults; home health care for persons entitled to SNF services; rural health clinic services; nurse-midwife services; and early and periodic screening, diagnosis, and treatment (EPSDT) for children.[42] States may also provide (and receive federal matching payments for) other services, including prescription drugs; dental care; eyeglasses; services provided by optometrists, podiatrists, and chiropractors; intermediate care facility (ICF) services; and services to the mentally retarded in ICFs. States vary considerably in the optional services they offer. Regardless of the services a state chooses to offer, it must do so uniformly throughout the state, providing comparable coverage to all categorically needy beneficiaries.

The required benefit package for the medically needy is less comprehensive. States opting to cover the medically needy must, at a minimum, furnish ambulatory care for children and prenatal care and delivery services for pregnant women. Almost all states that have medically needy programs, however, provide the same services to both medically and categorically needy recipients.

States have broad discretion in defining coverage for both mandatory and optional services. They may impose time or frequency limits on coverage, such as ceilings on inpatient days or physician visits. For example, in 1993, 49 states limited physicians' services to categorically needy beneficiaries in some ways.[43] They may establish utilization controls, such as medical necessity reviews, prior authorization for certain services, or second surgical opinion programs. Some states have instituted beneficiary cost-sharing as a form of utilization control. Federal statute constrains the use of this strategy, however, to nominal co-payments only (e.g., $1 per physician visit) and to certain groups of beneficiaries. Certain services, such as pregnancy and emergency care, are statutorily exempt from co-payment requirements.

Eligibility for Medicaid

Eligibility rules typically had been based on participation in cash assistance (welfare) programs. Because eligibility for these other programs can vary across states, so too does Medicaid eligibility. Most recent changes to federal eligibility rules have shifted from such program-based categories of eligibility to income-based definitions. The following discussion describes the evolution of current eligibility policies and the current composition of Medicaid beneficiaries.

Policies. As a means-tested entitlement program, eligibility for Medicaid was patterned after the earlier Kerr-Mills program and, until recently, has been closely linked to actual or potential receipt of cash assistance under various welfare programs. Persons qualified for coverage because they are either categorically needy or medically needy. Earlier, all persons receiving Aid to Families with Dependent Children (AFDC) and most persons on Supplemental Security Income (SSI) were considered categorically needy.[44] Certain groups not receiving cash assistance are also defined as categorically needy.[45]

From the passage of Medicaid in 1965 until the passage of welfare reform in the *Personal Responsibility and Work Opportunity Reconciliation Act* in 1996, Medicaid eligibility predominately was determined by welfare eligibility. Welfare reform eliminated the AFDC program. It, however, required states to provide Medicaid coverage to those who would have been previously eligible under AFDC rules. It also allowed states to expand Medicaid coverage to other low-income families. Welfare reform, however, has caused a drop in the number of people enrolled in Medicaid. Most states provided Medicaid eligibility to the medically needy. They are individuals whose income or resources exceed standards for cash assistance but who meet a separate state-determined income standard and are also aged, disabled, or a member of a family with dependent children. Persons who "spend down" income and assets due to large health-care expenses may qualify as medically needy.

Medicare Buy-in Arrangements. In contrast to Medicaid, Medicare is a national medical insurance program for the elderly and disabled. Several national requirements provide for Medicaid coverage of poor Medicare beneficiaries through state buy-in arrangements. State Medicaid programs serve Medicare beneficiaries in two distinct ways. First, they pay Medicare premiums and cost-sharing expenses for certain types of beneficiaries. In addition, they may provide benefits to those Medicare beneficiaries who qualify for the state's Medicaid program. In either case, Medicare is the primary insurer for these beneficiaries. The federal government partially reimburses states for their buy-in expenditures through the normal Medicaid grant formula.

Characteristics of those Covered by Medicaid

Medicaid recipients include a disproportionate share of females, non-whites, people living in poverty, the unemployed, young children, and central city dwellers. Children were four times more likely than adults to be on Medicaid.

Expenditure Patterns by Eligibility Category

Patterns of service use and overall expenditures differ dramatically among the three major populations served by Medicaid: children and adults in families, the elderly, and the disabled. Children and adults accounted for 73 percent of Medicaid beneficiaries in fiscal 1993, but only 31 percent of program payments.[46] By contrast, the elderly accounted for 33 percent of total payments, but only 12 percent of beneficiaries. Blind and disabled persons constituted 15 percent of beneficiaries, but accounted for 36 percent of payments. These differences are attributable largely to spending for long-term care for the elderly and disabled populations.[47]

Expenditures and Financing

Much of the criticism of the Medicaid program in the 1990s focused on rising expenditures. As the program is now structured, federal and state governments have difficulty controlling Medicaid spending.

Financing

States and the federal government jointly fund Medicaid. The federal share of expenditures is determined by a formula based on state per capita income, under which states with relatively low per capita incomes receive higher federal matching rates. For example, Mississippi, with a per capita income that is less than 70 percent of the national average, had a matching rate of about 79 percent, while Connecticut with a per capita income that is nearly 135 percent of the national average, received a 50 percent match.[48] Since 1987 this matching rate has been recalculated annually. Overall, federal funds accounted for about 57 percent of total Medicaid spending in 1995.

Federal payments to the states are provided from general revenues to match expenditures submitted by the states. There is no limit on the total amount of federal payments. States may finance their share entirely from state funds or require local governments to finance up to 60 percent of program costs. Only 14 states exercised the latter option in 1991, with local dollars accounting for a small proportion of state financing in most of these states.

Patterns in Program Spending

In 1966 spending for Medicaid and its predecessor, the Kerr-Mills medical assistance program, accounted for $1.5 billion or 3.7 percent of the nation's personal health-care expenditures.[49] By 1998, Medicaid's spending had increased to $170.6 billion and its share had climbed to about 16 percent of personal health-care expenditures in the United States. During this same period, the number of Medicaid beneficiaries grew from 12 to 36 million.[50] Recently, the number of enrollees and expenditures has been declining due to welfare reform.

In the early 1990s, state spending for Medicaid had been growing faster than any other category of state expenditures except for corrections. Its growth slowed in late 1990. Nevertheless, Medicaid accounts for about one-fifth of state expenditures and is the second largest category of state spending after elementary and secondary education. Medicaid spending differs dramatically by state, however. In 1993, the average annual payment per recipient of Medicaid services ranged from $2,381 in Mississippi to $9,700 in New Hampshire. The average spending per poor person ranged from $276 in Utah to $1,275 in the District of Columbia.[51]

While total state spending is a function of state population and the actual number of Medicaid beneficiaries, differences in service coverage, payment policies, and eligibility criteria are also contributing factors to spending differences across states. The pattern of Medicaid spending among service categories also varies by state. One state may put more money into long-term care, for example, while another state may emphasize inpatient hospital services.

Variation in states' total generosity for the Medicaid program is related to socio-economic factors, especially wealth and the federal matching rate.[52] Empirical evidence also suggests that states that are more generous in their funding for one aspect of Medicaid (e.g., eligibility, service coverage, and provider payments) tend to be less generous in others.[53]

Children's Health Insurance Program

The *Balanced Budget Act* of 1997 (BBA) included the State Children's Health Insurance Program (SCHIP). Congress authorized $24 billion expenditures over the five years in grants to states to provide health insurance for an estimated 2 to 4 million lower income children under SCHIP. All states and the District of Columbia have SCHIP programs. States have more flexibility in establishing eligibility, benefits, and cost-sharing for this program than for Medicaid.

Expenditures

Federal funds are allocated by two formulas, reflecting a political compromise. From 1998 to 2000, the distribution of funds to the states is based on the estimated number of uninsured children. After 2000, 75 percent of the formula will be based on the number of uninsured children and 25 percent on the number of low-income children.

States must match the federal expenditures. The match rate is a 30 percent enhancement of federal matching formula for Medicaid, but is capped at 85 percent of the total expenditures for each state.

Eligibility

Family income levels determine eligibility. Federal law establishes that uninsured children with incomes at or below 200 percent of poverty or 150 percent of state's Medicaid eligibility level, whichever is higher, are eligible. States can set their own eligibility levels below those levels, however. For example, states vary in their levels from under 133 percent of poverty to 300 percent of poverty.

A child covered by private insurance or Medicaid is not eligible for SCHIP. States must make efforts to avoid the "crowding out" of private insurance by this program. For example, California and Colorado enrol only children who have been uninsured for three months.[54]

Benefit Package

States can adopt one of three benefit packages for SCHIP: Medicaid, private plans, or a combination. Private plans must have benefits equivalent to the Federal Employees Blue Cross/Blue Shield Plan, coverage available to state employees, or coverage offered to the state's largest commercially enrolled population. Adoption of the Medicaid plan requires the state to provide full Medicaid benefits to SCHIP-covered children. Eighteen states and the District of Columbia are using Medicaid; 15 states are using private plans; and 17 states are using a combination of Medicaid and private plans.

If a state chooses to use private plans, those plans can charge nominal premiums and cost-sharing to children in families with incomes below 150 percent of the poverty line. For those children in families with incomes above 150 percent of poverty, cost-sharing and premiums can total up to a maximum of 5 percent of family income (except for preventive services which are exempt from cost-sharing). Those states that choose the Medicaid option cannot charge premiums.

Additional flexibility in SCHIP can be obtained by states. With waivers, states can enrol children in community-based health delivery systems, such as community health centres. States also can receive waivers to establish programs to cover entire families, if the costs are no more than for covering children alone.

Other Grant Programs

The Medicaid program dominates federal intergovernmental expenditures for health as well as for other areas. About one-third of all federal grant program expenditures are for Medicaid. It is the largest intergovernmental program. The other health programs are much smaller.

Other than Medicaid, smaller grant programs for general health, health-care services, and health research are authorized. Most of these programs are for specific projects; the remainder are determined by a formula with five of these being block grant programs. Most of the intergovernmental expenditures for health, however, are formula-based grants.

Regulation of Insurance

Constitutionally, the federal government could regulate health insurance (as well as other types of insurance) sold across state lines, but state governments conduct most regulation. Congress delegated authority to regulate insurance to the states in the *McCarran-Ferguson Act* of 1946. States monitor quality of care, financial solvency, consumer protection, fraud, dispute resolution, and marketing. Depending on the state, regulation is carried out by the state insurance commissioner, the state department of health or both. The type and degree of regulation varies dramatically by state.[55]

The federal government, however, has reasserted some jurisdiction over insurance. It controls quality, plan solvency, marketing for Medicare HMOs, and sets guidelines for state regulation for Medicaid HMOs. Major exceptions to state regulation of private insurance are contained in provisions of the *Employee Retirement Income Security Act* of 1974 (ERISA) and the *Health Insurance Portability and Accountability Act* of 1995 (HIPAA).

ERISA contains provisions that have caused intergovernmental conflicts. At its passage, its main purpose was to regulate solvency of retirement benefits, but it also applies to health benefits provided by employers. ERISA preempted all state laws related to employment benefits. It preserved the right of states to regulate insurance, but states could not deem employee plans to be insurance. These provisions have caused confusion. In general, employer-provided health plans which are self-insured cannot be regulated by states. Both state and federal governments regulate employer-purchased health insurance.[56] ERISA regulations do not cover the content of plans, but disclosure of information, administrative requirements, and fiduciary responsibility. Thus, Margaret Farrell concludes that "the effect ... has been to permit a largely unregulated market to define the health care available to the vast majority of Americans."[57] About 48 million people are in self-insured ERISA plans.[58]

There are two major areas of federal state conflict due to ERISA legislation. First, state health reform is difficult to implement, because courts have ruled based on ERISA that states cannot impose premium taxes, global budget enforcement, rating restrictions, and risk adjustments on self-insured health plans. Only Hawaii has an exemption to ERISA for its employer-mandated health insurance law, because it predated the passage of ERISA.[59] Second, conflicts are developing now over the inability of states to apply consumer protection provisions to ERISA plans.

The second major federal intervention in the private insurance market is HIPAA. Its purpose is to help those eligible individuals who change jobs or become unemployed to retain coverage by guaranteeing availability and renewability of insurance. HIPAA established limits on the use of pre-existing condition exclusions when someone changes plans in the group market. This provision, however, does not apply to the individual health insurance market. Second, HIPAA provides for guaranteed issue of insurance for qualified persons. Group insurers have to guarantee issue of all products to all small groups and to all eligible members of those groups. Finally, eligible individuals were guaranteed portability of coverage from group to individual insurance. Renewability of insurance is guaranteed in the individual market. It should be noted that these provisions do not assure affordability of insurance.[60] The Act imposes broad federal standards, but allows states to implement it in a flexible fashion. Although federal-state relationships vary by the specific provision of the law, generally HIPAA provides for minimum federal standards and partial preemption of state laws.[61] All states but three have passed their own laws to meet federal requirements. The secretary of health and human services enforces state compliance with the Act.[62] According to Kala Ladenheim, HIPAA is a "new template" for health-care relations between federal and state governments, threading "a narrow path between preemption and unfunded mandates."[63]

Other Regulation

State governments and voluntary organizations conduct regulation of health-care facilities and health professions. For example, physicians are licensed by states and those licences are generally only good in the issuing state. Specific medical boards grant specialty certification. Voluntary associations accredit medical education programs.

RECENT TRENDS

There has been a trend toward giving states more flexibility in grant programs and devolving more decision-making to the states.[64] In the Reagan administration, there were efforts to decentralize with creation of more block-grant programs and reductions in intergovernmental regulations. This trend was continued by the Clinton administration, but was heightened by the Republican Congress. The Clinton administration provided greater flexibility through the use of waivers of federal requirements in Medicaid and welfare programs. The *Balanced Budget Act* of 1997 provided more flexibility in Medicaid rules. As mentioned previously, legislation establishing a block-grant program to replace the categorical grant welfare program, which was established in the *Social Security Act* of 1935, was passed in 1996.[65] Congress also passed legislation to change Medicaid into a block-grant program, but President Clinton vetoed it. The State Children's Health Insurance Program was finally designed to be more flexible than traditional Medicaid.

Waivers

Provisions of the Medicaid law, such as the requirement that beneficiaries have the freedom to choose their providers, discouraged the development of managed care, while other provisions, such as federal eligibility standards, discouraged the use of federal moneys to broaden coverage to other populations in need of health insurance. States may obtain waivers of Medicaid requirements from the Health Care Financing Administration (HCFA), the federal agency that administers Medicaid, to address these concerns. There are different types of Medicaid waivers; these vary in the amount of flexibility allowed and in the provisions of the Medicaid law to which they apply. Two types of waivers are: program waivers under section 1915 of *the Social Security Act* and demonstration waivers granted under section 1115 of that Act.

Section 1915 allows HCFA to waive provisions of the Medicaid law so that states can mandate enrollment in managed care and develop home- and community-based care programs. HCFA can waive certain federal requirements (freedom of choice, uniform statewide operation, and comparability of benefits) to allow states to implement alternative health-delivery systems or provider reimbursement arrangements. To receive approval, a state must demonstrate that the program will be cost effective and that access to quality care will not be impaired. These waivers are granted for two years and can be renewed. Applications for these waivers are standardized. This is the most commonly used waiver authority.

Section 1115(a) of the *Social Security Act* allows the secretary of health and human services (HHS) to approve demonstration projects that will help promote the goals of the Medicaid program. States have used section 1115 authority to expand eligibility for Medicaid to include the uninsured and to enrol beneficiaries in managed care. The intent of this demonstration authority is to test unique and innovative approaches to the delivery and financing of health care. Demonstrations require research and evaluation components. In contrast to section 1915 waivers, states are not allowed merely to copy programs in other states to obtain approval for demonstration authority. Nevertheless, under the Clinton administration, the federal government appeared to be willing to approve waiver requests that were only slightly different than previously approved ones. The secretary has broad discretion in approving these demonstrations and has selectively approved such proposals. For example, while the Oregon demonstration proposal, which included expanded eligibility and priority-setting for health-care benefits, was rejected because of concerns about its implications for the *Americans with Disabilities Act*, a modified proposal was later approved. These demonstrations are for a limited time, usually three to five years. The HHS secretary generally has not renewed them, but Congress has extended them with legislation. From 1984 to 1991, Congress legislated 13 extensions of demonstration waivers.[66]

In January 1997, HCFA had approved section 1915b waivers in 42 states.[67] By 1998, 16 states had implemented section 1115 waivers and an additional two had received section 1115 waivers, but had not implemented them.

Block Grants

There have been significant proposals to turn Medicaid into a block-grant program. These would provide the states with more flexibility in running their programs, especially in service delivery and payment mechanisms, and would reduce national expenditures on Medicaid.

A proposal passed by Congress in November 1995 (H.R. 2491), but vetoed by President Clinton would have changed Medicaid into a block-grant program (referred to as a Medigrant). Under the block-grant approach, states would have received a set amount of federal funds to use in providing health-care services to people with incomes below some threshold. In general, states would have been able to decide which groups of poor people to cover and what services to provide them. Eligibility would have been changed under the Medigrant proposal. Each state would have decided who among those under 275 percent of the poverty line would be eligible for its Medigrant program. While eligibility entitlement for groups of individuals would have been eliminated, states would have been required to cover pregnant women or children under 13 with family incomes below the poverty level as well as disabled individuals as defined by the states. Additionally, money would have to be set aside for specific groups. States would have been required to spend at least 85 percent of the average percentages they allocated previously for each of the following groups: poor families, low-income elderly beneficiaries, and low-income disabled individuals.

As for most other aspects, the Medigrant proposal would have allowed states considerable flexibility to design their programs. They would have had complete freedom to select specific services to be provided (except for abortion), set the level of payments, vary benefits by types of individuals and geographic areas, and determine use of managed care.

Unfunded Mandates

In 1995 the *Unfunded Mandates Act* was passed. It provided that any act with state and local cost implications over $50 million could be stopped by a point of order raised in either house of Congress. Although a majority of the legislative body could overrule the point of order, it provides for an opportunity for consideration of the mandate. The power of this legislation appears to be in preempting legislative developments, not in stopping them on the floor of the House or Senate.[68]

EFFECTIVENESS

During my lifetime, there have been several crises of federalism and dramatic changes in intergovernmental relations. Since the mid-1940s, we have moved from a grant system that included about 30 programs (distributing under $900 million) to over 600 programs (distributing over $225 billion). But that overall trend hides more recent developments. Since the Reagan administration, there has been a trend toward decentralization.[69]

There have been many efforts in the last 50 years to revise our federal system. President Richard Nixon proposed that a national standard income for families under his Family Assistance Plan replace the state-administered welfare system. His political descendants, however, recently decentralized welfare. Under another proposal, Alice Rivlin, a Democratic political officeholder, proposed giving federal programs in housing, social services, and education to the states. Programs that need uniformity (social insurance and health insurance) would become national programs, according to Rivlin.[70] As can be seen easily, there are no generally accepted principles concerning the division of responsibility in the United States.[71] Division of responsibility is a political solution, ever evolving.

Federal-State Conflicts

Recently, there have been conflicts between federal and state governments over Medicaid. First, concerns over Medicaid are part of the general concerns over the grant system. As part of that general concern, states are troubled with what they see as federal mandates in the Medicaid program. Second, according to states, Medicaid does not provide enough flexibility in program design to respond to local conditions. Third, growth in Medicaid expenditures exacerbated the relationship between federal and state governments. Finally, states and their supporters have claimed that decision-making has shifted to the federal government. Many of these concerns have been alleviated with the passage of the *Balanced Budget Act* of 1997 and a very good economy, however.

Mandates

States and their supporters have been dissatisfied with the dramatic growth of grant programs as well as with increasing conditions for receiving grants. The Advisory Commission on Intergovernmental Relations (ACIR) argued that "if there has been a single phenomena which has worked ... to erode the concept of federalism, it has been the dramatic expansion in the number, scope, and purpose of federal grants in aid."[72] David Walker, a former director of the ACIR, has described our federal system as being overloaded. The overload was caused by a deluge of federal programs and dollars since the 1960s, funding for all governmental entities (not merely states), states having subordinate positions in many grant programs, creeping conditionalism for grants, and provision of grants to quasi-governmental institutions.[73]

Since the 1990s there has been a growing concern with unfunded mandates as conditions for federal grant programs. According to Fix and Kenyon, unfunded mandates include direct orders with criminal or civil penalties, cross-program requirements, and cross-program sanctions.[74] Mandates skew the use of state resources and place an inappropriate weight on federal decision-making. The *Unfunded Mandates Reform Act* of 1995 (P.L. 104-4) required the ACIR to examine mandates which "(1) require state or local governments to expend substantial amounts of their own resources without regard for state and local priorities; (2) abridge historical powers of state and local governments without a clear showing of national need; (3) impose requirements that are difficult or impossible to implement; and (4) are the subject of widespread objections."

The only health-care mandate identified by the ACIR was the Boren Amendment. It required states to establish Medicaid payment rates for hospitals, nursing home facilities, and intermediate care facilities that are "reasonable and adequate to meet the costs which must be incurred by efficiently and economically operated facilities."[75] Ironically, the Boren Amendment was passed originally to give the states more flexibility in setting payments. Prior federal law required that payment be determined on the basis of reasonable costs. The Boren Amendment does not meet the definition of mandates as set forth by Fix and Kenyon: it did not involve direct orders with civil or criminal penalties, cross-program requirements or sanctions. It was merely a condition of participation in the program. Nevertheless, the Boren Amendment was a problem for states because it gave interest groups a tool to challenge payment rates at a time of increased health-care costs.[76] In Pennsylvania, Washington, and Virginia, Medicaid payment rates were increased in response to court decisions based on the Boren Amendment.[77] The *Balanced Budget Act* of 1997 repealed the Boren Amendment.

Flexibility

The ACIR and others complained that the Medicaid program was not flexible enough to accommodate local differences and needs.[78] For example, there has been tension between federal requirements regarding freedom of choice and states' desire to use managed care to limit growth in expenditures. The *Balanced Budget Act*, however, made numerous changes including allowing the states without waivers to require Medicaid beneficiaries to enrol in managed-care organizations that serve only Medicaid recipients. Beneficiaries, except for children with special needs, Medicare recipients, and Indians, can be locked into a specific health plan for a year.

SCHIP and HIPAA provide more flexibility than does Medicaid. Indeed, the Reforming States Group, a voluntary group of health policy leaders had recommended that future health programs have broad federal standards and state implementation like SCHIP and HIPAA.[79]

Expenditures

The pressure of Medicaid expenditures on state budgets was a source of tension in our intergovernmental system. The ACIR, for example, complained that state costs increased due to unilateral changes in program requirements made by the federal government.[80] Scholarly studies, however, have shown that there were multiple factors causing state expenditure growth.[81] In judging state complaints about federal influence on state budgets, we have to remember that roughly 60 percent of all Medicaid spending is for services and beneficiaries that are not required by federal law.[82]

Many state officials argue that the Medicaid program spending crowds out state spending for other services. In one of the few academic studies of this issue, Fossett and Wyckoff concluded that Medicaid spending had little effect on educational spending in states.[83]

Federal Influence

According to the ACIR, Medicaid decision-making shifted disproportionately to the federal government.[84] This complaint is hard to substantiate or refute. Indeed, as evidence, the ACIR could only cite changes that cost the states money.[85] States, however, were effective in shifting costs to the federal government with the use of provider taxes and gifts from providers. For example, Pennsylvania hospitals formed a foundation, borrowed money, and donated it to the state for Medicaid expenditures. The federal government matched expenditures for those donated funds, which were then used to reimburse the borrowed money.[86]

Absolute federal control is a myth. State and local officials help shape the development and implementation of policies.[87] For example, since the 1930s federal standards for welfare included statewide uniformity in program, and professionalism in administration. Massachusetts' tradition of local, unprofessional welfare delivery ran counter to this provision. It was not until the mid-1960s that Massachusetts complied with those federal standards established in the 1930s.[88] Grant programs reflect the individual state political cultures. But more importantly, states are free to refuse to adopt grant programs.

Policy Variation across States

There is little uniformity in the Medicaid program. There are variations in the populations covered, services delivered, and expenditures made across states. Eligibility and benefits are based on state residency. These differences are determined by the wealth of the states (even though the grant formula favours poor states) and, to some extent, their politics.[89]

Variation across the states can cause problems. In welfare policy, Peterson and Rom have shown that states with generous benefits are welfare magnets, attracting or retaining the poor.[90] Since states do not want to attract poor people but the wealthy, they limit the generosity of welfare policies.

One of the longest recognized problems, the matching formula, is not a source of tension with all states, but affects states differently. It does not effectively target need.[91] The matching formula is based on per capita income with those states with lower per capita income receiving a higher federal match ratio. The ACIR recommended that the formula include state fiscal capacity, while the GAO recommended the use of state taxable resources and people in poverty. But even with a change in the formula, it is likely that wealthy states will spend more on the poor, because they can afford to do that.

Rationality

The pattern of grants is not rational in an economic sense, but has its roots in the political institutions.[92] Phillip Monypenny wrote "federal aid programs are an outcome of a loose coalition which resorts to a mixed federal-state program because it is not strong enough in individual states to secure its program, and because it is not united enough to be able to achieve a wholly federal program against the opposition which a specific program would engender."[93] Requirements of particular programs, including Medicaid, are a result of the efforts of loose coalitions over time.

Part of our lack of rationality in program development does not lie in our federal system, but in our party system and government. Our political parties are loose coalitions without core goals and with few mechanisms for control. Candidates owe little allegiance to parties. Separation of powers between legislative, executive, and judicial branches of government, our most fundamental principle, makes the development of rational intergovernmental policies futile. What is rational, in the US context, is what works. As Monypenny wrote, "The grant-in-aid system is by no means an undermining of federalism, but rather a refinement of it. It corresponds to a pragmatic pluralism, which has long been remarked as a characteristic of politics in the United States."[94]

CONCLUSIONS

There is continuous change in the balance between the power and roles of the federal and state governments in health policy and other areas. Our first Chief Justice of the Supreme Court, John Marshall, noted that the question about the extent of federal power "is perpetually arising, and will probably continue to arise, as long as our system shall exist."[95]

NOTES

I would like to thank Daniel Fox and Steven Schroeder for their comments on this paper. The views expressed in this chapter are those of the author and do not necessarily reflect those of the Robert Wood Johnson Foundation.

[1]Alexander Hamilton, John Jay and James Madison, *The Federalist* (New York: The Modern Library, n.d.), p. 249.

[2]Thomas J. Anton, *American Federalism and Public Policy* (New York: Random House, 1989), p. 9.

[3]*McClulloch v. Maryland*, 4 Wheaton 316 (1819).

[4]Hamilton, Jay and Madison, *The Federalist*, p. 268.

[5]*U.S. v. Butler*, 297 U.S. 1 (1936).

[6]*Gibbons v. Ogden*, 9 Wheaton 1 (1824).

[7]*Cooley v. The Board of Wardens of Philadelphia*, 12 Howard 99 (1852).

[8]*Paul v. Virginia*, 8 Wall 168 (1869).

[9]*U.S. v. South-Eastern Underwriters Association,* 322 U.S. 533 (1944).

[10]*Jacobson v. Commonwealth of Massachusetts*, 197 U.S. 11 (1905).

[11]*Garcia v. San Antonio Metropolitan Transit Authority*, 469 U.S. 528 (1985).

[12]*U.S. v. Lopez 514* U.S. 549(1995).

[13]John Kincaid, "Intergovernmental Deregulation?" *Public Administration Review* 55 (September/October 1955):495.

[14]*Seminole Tribe of Florida v. U.S.* 517 U.S. 44 (1996); *Printz v. U.S.* 521 U.S. 898 (1997); *Alden v. Maine* 527 U.S. 706 (1999).

[15]David B.Walker, *Toward a Functioning Federalism* (Cambridge, MA: Winthrop Publishers, 1981).

[16]John Shannon and James Edwin Kee, "The Rise of Competitive Federalism," *Public Budgeting and Finance* 9 (Winter 1989):5-20.

[17]*Commonwealth of Massachusetts v. Mellon*, 262 U.S. 447 (1923).

[18]*Commonwealth of Massachusetts v. Mellon*, 262 U.S. 447 (1923).

[19]For example, concerning federal grants for highways, see *State of Oklahoma v. U.S. Civil Service Commission,* 330 U.S. 127 (1947).

[20]Barbara G. Rosenkrantz, *Public Health and the State: Changing Views in Massachusetts, 1842-1936* (Cambridge, MA: Harvard University Press, 1972), p. 154.

[21]Rosemary Stevens, *American Medicine and the Public Interest* (New Haven: Yale University Press, 1971); Edward R. Schlesinger, "The Sheppard-Towner Era: A Prototype Case Study in Federal State Relationships," *American Journal of Public Health* 56 (June 1967):1034-41.

[22]*Steward v. Davis*, 301 U.S. 548 (1937).

[23]Robert Stevens and Rosemary Stevens, *Welfare Medicine in America* (New York: Free Press, 1974).

[24]For a discussion of this point, see John Harrigan, *Politics and Policy in State and Communities* (Boston: Little, Brown and Company, 1980).

[25]Paul Fronstin, "Trends in Employment-Based Health Benefits," Presentation, 6 May 1998, Washington, DC.

[26]For a good description of local market variations, see Paul B. Ginsburg and Nancy J. Fasciano, *The Community Snapshots Project: Capturing Health System Change* (Washington, DC: Center for Studying Health System Change, 1996).

[27]Robert F. Rich and William D. White, *Health Policy, Federalism, and the American States* (Washington, DC: Urban Institute, 1996), p. 18.

[28]United States, Advisory Commission on Intergovernmental Relations (ACIR), *Public Assistance: The Growth of a Federal System* (Washington, DC: ACIR, 1980).

[29]Martha Derthick, *The Influence of Federal Grants: Public Assistance in Massachusetts* (Cambridge, MA: Harvard University Press, 1970).

[30]Katherine Levit, Cathy Cowan, Bradley Braden, Jean Stiller, Arthur Sensenig and Helen Lazenby, "National Health Expenditures in 1997: More Slow Growth," *Health Affairs* 17 (November/December 1998):99-110.

[31]Sheila Smith, Mark Freeland, Stephen Heffler, David McKusick, "The Next Ten Years of Health Spending: What Does the Future Hold?" *Health Affairs* 17 (September/October 1998):129.

[32]Sylvia Law, *Blue Cross: What Went Wrong* (New Haven: Yale University Press, 1974).

[33]Paul Starr, *The Transformation of American Medicine* (New York: Basic Books, 1982), pp. 295-97.

[34]US House of Representatives, Committee on Ways and Means, *1998 Green Book* (Washington, DC: Government Printing Office, 1998).

[35]Ibid., p. 838.

[36]Medicare Payment Advisory Commission, *Health Care Spending and the Medicare Program: A Data Book* (Washington, DC: MedPAC,1998):20.

[37]Paul Fronstin, "Nonelderly Americans' Insurance Status," *EBRI Notes* 19 (November 1998):1-5.

[38]Phillip Cooper and Barbara Steinberg Shone, "More Offers, Fewer Takers for Employment-Based Health Insurance: 1987 and 1996," *Health Affairs* 16 (November/December 1997):142-56.

[39]Physician Payment Review Commission, *Annual Report to Congress 1997* (Washington, DC: PPRC, 1997):318-19.

[40]American Hospital Association, *Hospital Statistics* (Chicago, IL: Hospital Forum, 1999), pp. 4-5.

[41]American Medical Association, *Physician Characteristics and Distribution in the U.S.* (Chicago, IL: AMA, 1999).

[42]Eligibility categories are discussed below. The categorically needy are generally those who receive welfare benefits.

[43]United States, Department of Health and Human Services, Health Care Financing Administration, *Medicaid State Profile Data System: Characteristics of Medicaid State Programs*, Vol. 1 (Baltimore, MD:HCFA, 1993).

[44]Twelve states exercise the more restrictive 209(b) option by limiting Medicaid eligibility for SSI beneficiaries to more restrictive standards that were in effect in the state before implementation of SSI.

[45]These include (i) persons whose cash payments would be less than $10, (ii) families that lose AFDC benefits due to increased employment income, working hours, or child or special support payments, (iii) persons who become ineligible for SSI due to increases in their Social Security benefits, (iv) disabled persons who lose SSI due to employment income but who remain disabled and need Medicaid benefits to stay employed, and (v) children receiving federal adoption assistance or foster care maintenance payments.

[46]Disproportionate share hospital expenditures are made to those hospitals that serve a disproportionate number of low-income patients.

[47]United States, Congress, Congressional Research Service, *Medicaid Source Book: Background Data and Analysis* (Washington, DC: Government Printing Office, 1988).

[48]The federal match for Medicaid services is legislatively set at a minimum of 50 percent and maximum of 83 percent. Program administration costs are matched at 50 percent, and higher matching rates are provided for data systems operations and quality monitoring efforts.

[49]Helen Lazenby, Katherine R. Levit and Daniel R. Waldo, "National Health Expenditures, 1985," *Health Care Financing Notes* 6 (September 1986):1-32. The Kerr-Mills program provided grants for medical care furnished to the low-income elderly. Although the program had the potential to extend services to a substantial proportion of the elderly population, it was viewed primarily as a supplement to existing forms of public assistance and as a means to shift the burden of financing to the federal government. Medicaid expanded and replaced the Kerr-Mills program (Stevens and Stevens, *Welfare Medicine in America*.

[50]Cathy Cowan, Helen C. Lazenby, Anne B. Martin, Patricia A. McDonnell, Arthur L. Sensenig, Jean M. Stiller, Lekha S. Whittle, Kimberly A. Kotova, Mark A. Zezza, Carolyn S. Donham, Anna M. Long and Madie W. Stewart, "National Health Expenditures, 1998," *Health Care Financing Review* 21 (Winter 1999):165-210.

[51]David Liska, Karen Obermaier, Barbara Lyons, and Peter Lang, *Medicaid Expenditures and Beneficiaries: National and State Profiles and Trends* (Washington, DC: Kaiser Commission on the Future of Medicaid, 1995).

[52]Stephen Davidson, *Medicaid Decisions: A Systematic Analysis of the Cost Problem* (Cambridge, MA: Ballinger, 1980); Thomas W. Grannemann, "Reforming National Health Programs for the Poor," in *National Health Insurance: What Now, What Later? What Never?*, ed. Mark V. Pauly (Washington, DC: American Enterprise Institute, 1980); John Holahan and Joel W. Cohen, *Medicaid: The Tradeoff between Cost Containment and Access to Care* (Washington, DC: Urban Institute Press, 1986); Robert J. Buchanan, Joseph C. Capelleri and Robert L. Ohlsfeldt, "The Social Environment and Medicaid Expenditures: Factors Influencing the Level of State Medicaid Spending, *Public Administration Review* 51 (January/February 1991):67-73.

[53]Jerry Cromwell, Sylvia Hurdle and Rachel Schurman, "Defederalizing Medicaid: Fair to the Poor, Fair to Taxpayers?" *Journal of Health Politics, Policy and Law* 12,1 (Spring 1987):1-34.

[54]United States, National Economic Council and Domestic Policy Council, "Implementation of the Children's Health Insurance Program: Six Month Progress Report," 1 April 1998.

[55]For a discussion of variation in state regulation of quality, see Physician Payment Review Commission, *Annual Report to Congress 1995* (Washington, DC: PPRC, 1996), pp. 344-49.

[56]For a description of the politics of the passage of ERISA, see Daniel M. Fox and Daniel C. Schaffer, "Health Policy and ERISA: Interest Groups and Semipreemption," *Journal of Health Politics, Policy and Law* 14 (Summer 1989):239-60.

[57]Margaret Farrell, "ERISA Preemption and Regulation of Managed Health Care: The Case for Managed Federalism," *American Journal of Law and Medicine* 23 (1997):265.

[58]Craig Copeland and Bill Pierron, "Implications of ERISA for Health Benefits and the Number of Self-Funded ERISA Plans," *The Future of Health Benefits: EBRI-ERF Policy Forum*, 6 May 1998, pp. 71 -94.

[59]Physician Payment Review Commission, *Annual Report to Congress 1995*, pp. 414-19.

[60]Beth C. Fuchs, Bob Lyke, Richard Price and Madeleine Smith, "The Health Insurance Portability and Accountability Act of 1996: Guidance on Frequently Asked Questions," *CRS Report for Congress*, Congressional Research Service, 10 April 1997.

[61]Kala Ladenheim, "Health Insurance in Transition: The Health Insurance Portability and Accountability Act of 1966," *Publius* 27 (Spring 1997):33-51.

[62]Len M. Nichols and Linda J. Blumberg, "A Different Kind of 'New Federalism'? The Health Insurance Portability and Accountability Act of 1996," *Health Affairs* 17 (May/June 1998):25-42.

[63]Ladenheim, "Health Insurance in Transition."

[64]For a more comprehensive history of this, see Frank J. Thompson and John J. Dilulio (eds.), *Medicaid and Devolution: A View from the States* (Washington, DC: The Brookings Institution, 1998).

[65]For a description of welfare block grant, see Irene Lurie, "Temporary Assistance for Needy Families," *Publius: The Journal of Federalism* 27 (Spring 1997):73-87.

[66]Congressional Research Service, *Medicaid Source Book: Background Data and Analysis* (Washington, DC: Government Printing Office, 1993).

[67]Andy Schneider,"Overview of Medicaid Managed Care Provisions in the Balanced Budget Act of 1997," paper prepared for the Kaiser Commission on the Future of Medicaid, December 1997.

[68]Paul L. Posner, "Unfunded Mandates Reform Act: 1996 and Beyond," *Publius: The Journal of Federalism* 27 (Spring 1997):53-71.

[69]John Chubb, "Federalism and the Bias for Centralization," in *The New Direction in American Politics*, ed. John E. Chubb and Paul E. Peterson (Washington, DC: The Brookings Institution, 1985), pp. 273-306.

[70]Alice M. Rivlin, *Reviving the American Dream: The Economy, the States and the Federal Government* (Washington, DC: The Brookings Institution, 1992).

[71]Mark V. Pauly, "Income Redistribution as a Local Public Good," *Journal of Public Economics* 2 (February 1978):35-58; Helen F. Ladd and Fred C. Doolittle, "Which Level of Government Should Assist the Poor?" *National Tax Journal* 35 (September 1982):323-36.

[72]United States, Advisory Commission on Intergovernmental Relations, *Public Assistance*, p. 91.

[73]Walker, *Toward a Functioning Federalism*.

[74]Michael Fox and Daphne Kenyon (eds.), *Coping with Mandates: What are the Alternatives* (Washington, DC: Urban Institute, 1990).

[75]United States, Advisory Commission on Intergovernmental Relations, *The Role of Federal Mandates in Intergovernment Relations* (Washington, DC: ACIR, 1996) (Preliminary Report), p. 9.

[76]Barbara Booling Manard, "Repeal of the Boren Amendment: Background, Implications, and Next Steps" (Washington, DC: Georgetown Medical Center, 1997, unpublished paper).

[77]Gerald Anderson and William Scanlon, "Medicaid Payment Policy and the Boren Amendment," in *Medicaid Financing Crisis: Balancing Responsibilities, Priorities and Dollars*, ed. Diane Rowland, Judith Feder and Alina Salganicoff (Washington, DC: American Association for the Advancement of Science Press, 1993), pp. 83-94.

[78]United States, Advisory Commission on Intergovernmental Relations, *Medicaid: Intergovernmental Trends and Options* (Washington, DC: ACIR, 1992).

[79]The Reforming States Group, "Balanced Federalism and Health System Reform," *Health Affairs* 17 (May/June 1998):181-91..

[80]Advisory Commission on Intergovernmental Relations, *Medicaid*.

[81]Stephen Long, "Causes of Soaring Medicaid Spending, 1988-1991," in *Medicaid Financing Crisis*, ed. Rowland, Feder and Salganicoff, pp. 1-21; John Holahan,Teresa Coughlin, Leighton Ku, David Heslam and Colin Winterbottom, "Understanding the Recent Growth in Medicaid Spending," in *Medicaid Financing Crisis*, ed. Rowland, Feder and Salganicoff, pp. 23-42.

[82]Diane Rowland, "Medicaid's Role," Testimony, Subcommittee on Health and the Environment, US House of Representatives, Commerce Committee, 11 March 1997.

[83]James W. Fossett and James H. Wyckoff, "Has Medicaid Growth Crowded Out State Educational Spending," *Journal of Health Politics, Policy and Law* 21 (Fall 1996):409-32.

[84]Advisory Commission on Intergovernmental Relations, *Medicaid*.

[85]Ibid.

[86]For example, see US General Accounting Office (GAO), *Medicaid: States Use Illusory Approaches to Shift Program Cost to Federal Government* (Washington, DC: GAO, 1994).

[87]Thomas J. Anton, "New Federalism and Intergovernmental Fiscal Relationships: The Implications for Health Policy," *Journal of Health Politics, Policy and Law* 22 (June 1977):690-720. Phillip Monypenny, David C. Colby and David G. Baker, "The Politics of Legislative Interference in Certificate of Need Decisions," *Journal of Health and Human Resources Administration* 5 (Spring 1983):409-26.

[88]Derthick, *The Influence of Federal Grants.*

[89]Charles J.Barrilleaux and Mark E. Miller, "The Political Economy of State Medicaid Policy," *American Political Science Review* 82 (December 1988):1089-107.

[90]Paul E. Peterson and Mark C. Rom, *Welfare Magnets: A New Case for National Standards* (Washington, DC: The Brookings Institution, 1990).

[91]US General Accounting Office, *Medicaid: Alternatives for Improving the Distribution of Funds* (Washington, DC: GAO, 1991); Advisory Commission on Intergovernmental Relations, *Medicaid.*

[92]Phillip Monypenny, "Federal Grants-in-Aid to State Governments: A Political Analysis," *National Tax Journal* 13 (March 1960):1-16; John E. Chubb, "Federalism and the Bias for Centralization," in *The New Direction in American Politics*, ed. Chubb and Peterson, pp. 273-306.

[93]Monypenny, "Federal Grants-in-Aid to State Governments: A Political Analysis," p. 16.

[94]Ibid.

[95]*McClulloch v. Maryland*, 4 Wheaton 316 (1819).

6

FEDERALISM AND HEALTH CARE IN CANADA

Antonia Maioni

Canada's system of government is a federal one but, as many comparative scholars have noted, all federal systems do not work in the same way. Federalism typically involves the allocation of jurisdictional responsibilities such as policy-making among different levels of government.[1] One ideal type of federalism portrays the division of powers between governments as independent "watertight compartments," another as more "coordinate" in nature.[2] In the real world of Canadian federalism, power is formally divided between the federal government and the provinces, but in many important policy sectors both levels of government are responsible for ensuring the well-being of citizens.

The discussion in this chapter focuses on how Canadian federalism has shaped one of the most important policy sectors of the modern welfare state, namely health care. The federal-provincial relationship has had a profound impact on the emergence, and subsequent development, of health-care provision and financing in Canada. While primary jurisdiction for health care lies in the policy domain of the provincial governments, the federal government now occupies an important financial and political space in the health arena.

THE CONSTITUTIONAL FRAMEWORK

The division of powers enumerated in the *Constitution Acts* of 1867 and 1982 set the parameters of the federal arrangement in Canada. These statutes reveal

a tension between a centralizing tendency implied in the economic and residual powers allocated to the federal government, and the decentralizing effect
of the wide-ranging responsibilities accorded to the provinces. This tension
has been exacerbated since 1867 by a variety of factors, including judicial
interpretations favouring the provinces and the passage of the 1982 Charter of
Rights and Freedoms. Nevertheless, periods of intergovernmental cooperation
did lead to important policy initiatives, including the programs that form the
core of the welfare state in Canada.

Health care is a prime example of this dynamic. There were few specific
references to health care in *Constitution Act, 1867*, but conflict between levels
of government intensified with the growth of the public role in the sector. In
1867, health concerns were considered private rather than public matters, within
the bounds of family responsibility and charitable institutions or religious communities, and government intervention was primarily limited to matters of public
health.[3] As the responsibilities of the modern state expanded over time, the
enumeration of provincial responsibilities yielded a wider interpretation in the
health sector. Section 92(7) of the *Constitution Act* allows provincial legislatures to enact laws for the "Establishment, Maintenance, and Management of
Hospitals, Asylums, Charities and Eleemosynary Institutions," and section
92(16) gives provincial legislatures jurisdiction over "Generally all Matters of
a merely local or private Nature in the Province." In addition, the courts have
held that insurance falls within the provincial domain, a position established
most clearly with the invalidation of the *Employment and Social Insurance Act*
of 1935 on the grounds that it went beyond the power of the federal government.

Despite the fact that, formally speaking, health policy is considered to
be primarily within the bounds of provincial jurisdiction, the federal government also occupies an important political space in the sector. Part of this space
is related to the federal government's constitutional responsibilities for public
health matters under section 91(11) and for the general welfare of specific
classes of people such as "Indians," "aliens," inmates in federal prisons and
members of the armed forces. More important, however, is the fiscal power of
the federal government. Although the federal government cannot legislate directly in provincial health systems, it does have broad taxing powers at its
disposal, such as the provisions of section 91(3) for the "raising of Money by
any Mode or System of Taxation." Fiscal power has given the federal government considerable policy leverage. The modern interpretation of the federal
government's role can be traced to the 1940 Report of the Royal Commission
on Dominion-Provincial Relations, which claimed that, because of the heavy

financial burden imposed by social programs,the federal government could assist the provinces through cost-sharing or fiscal transfers.[4] Consequently, the federal government has developed the doctrine of a "spending power," which allows it to spend revenues outside its formal areas of jurisdiction.

While the federal government's involvement in health care has been primarily confined to the use of the federal spending power, the allocation of money has an obvious impact on provincial health policy. Two examples of the federal spending power are relevant for health care. The first is the use of transfer payments, whereby federal funds are used to pay part of the costs of a provincial program. Examples include the original shared-cost programs in hospital and medical insurance, as well as subsequent block-funding arrangements, such as the Established Programs Financing (EPF) which funded health care and postsecondary education after 1976 and the Canada Health and Social Transfer (CHST) which has covered health, education, and social assistance since 1995. The second major federal spending instrument is equalization payments. These payments are not targeted directly at specific programs, but rather are unconditional transfers to less well-off provinces. The rationale for equalization payments is to assist provinces with less powerful economies in providing similar levels of health care and other services to their populations.

These transfers produce very different patterns of support in various provinces. In the Atlantic provinces, federal funds account for almost 40 percent of provincial revenues; in the richer provinces, they account for less than 20 percent of revenues. There is also a significant difference in the balance between CHST and equalization grants, and therefore between tied and untied funds, across the provinces. Of the total federal revenues allocated to the provinces for 1999–2000, 71 percent flowed through the CHST, while 23 percent were in the form of equalization payments. The less well-off the province, however, the higher the ratio of equalization to CHST payments: for example, only 36 percent of federal transfers to Newfoundland are distributed through the CHST while for Quebec the figure is 63 percent, and for the three richest provinces it is100 percent (see Table 1). Although the rationale for the deployment of the federal sending power is to ensure that all Canadians, regardless of province of residence, enjoy similar health and social benefits, many provinces have expressed dissatisfaction with federal involvement. Richer provinces such as Alberta, British Columbia, and Ontario have chafed under the redistributive burdens of the equalization program, while successive Quebec governments have contended that the federal government should not interfere in areas of exclusive provincial jurisdiction.

TABLE 1
Federal Fiscal Transfers to the Provinces, 1998
($millions)

	CHST	Equalization
Newfoundland	510	1,088
Prince Edward Island	117	328
Nova Scotia	816	1,301
New Brunswick	647	1,093
Quebec	6,895	4,820
Ontario	9,253	0
Manitoba	975	1,016
Saskatchewan	850	117
Alberta	2,236	0
British Columbia	1,574	0

Source: Canada. Department of Finance, *Federal Transfers to Provinces and Territories* (Ottawa: Supply and Services Canada, 1999).

Canadian federalism is also characterized by the absence of effective institutional representation for the provinces within the federal government. Apart from the tradition of regional representation within the federal Cabinet and the largely symbolic functions of an appointed Senate, there is no legal role for provincial governments in the formation and passage of federal legislation. In the absence of such formal institutions, other intergovernmental mechanisms have developed to allow for the exchange of information and to coordinate policy-making. Executive federalism refers to the process of "federal-provincial diplomacy" between the political executives of the two orders of government, which takes place in a variety of settings. Most important are First Ministers' Conferences (FMC), at which the Canadian prime minister and provincial premiers discuss major policy issues. Federal and provincial ministers in specific policy areas such as health also meet regularly, and the provincial premiers gather annually without their federal counterpart. (Quebec does not always officially attend these meetings although representatives are usually present as observers.) In addition to these "executive" level exchanges, there are hundreds of administrative intergovernmental committees engaged in coordinating federal-provincial programs and the exercise of fiscal federalism. Both the FMC and the more specialized meetings of ministers and officials are designed to air grievances in certain policy areas or to propose new initiatives. Although these meetings are often major political events in themselves, they do not always succeed in resolving intergovernmental conflict, nor do they impose any restraints on the federal government's ability to make unilateral decisions about the use of its spending power.

Regional representation at the federal level has also been affected by the political party system. Originally a two-party system of "national" parties, party politics in Canada is now characterized by the presence of regional parties in the House of Commons and provincial legislatures that do not reflect the same mix of parties. In addition, party organizations and platforms at the federal and provincial levels are not necessarily harmonized. Regional opposition parties in the House of Commons, such as the Canadian Alliance and the Bloc Québécois, argue for more decentralization in the Canadian federation, albeit for different reasons. Strong provincial parties, such as the Conservative party in Alberta and Ontario and the Parti Québécois in Quebec, express dissatisfaction with the way in which federal decisions affect their policy-making capacities. Despite these conflicts, it should be remembered that the rise of regional parties and the presence of disciplined parties within centralized parliamentary structures did much to facilitate the development of the welfare state in Canada, in particular comprehensive programs such as health insurance.[5]

THE HEALTH-CARE SYSTEM IN CANADA

In terms of both popularity and money spent, health care represents the most impressive piece of social policy in Canada. A consensus has developed that health care, and more specifically affordable access to quality care, is a public good which both levels of government have a responsibility in maintaining. Health care has escaped much of the backlash directed at other social programs, such as social assistance or unemployment insurance, and it is unlikely governments could disengage themselves from the health-care sector as surreptitiously as has been the case with family allowances, for example. The reasons for this include the obvious: because health care is a universal program and a service provided to individuals rather than a direct transfer based on income, much of the controversy associated with redistribution is absent in debates over health-care reform; and provincial health-care systems, despite their financial woes and delivery problems, have successfully provided quality care based on need for all residents at a comparatively reasonable cost. In comparison with other industrialized countries, Canada spends a relatively high proportion of its gross domestic product on health care; per capita expenditure levels also place Canada in the top tier of health-care spenders (see Table 2). But the country has been relatively successful in containing health-care costs in the past decade, even considering the fact that the ratio of private to public expenditures has increased. Overall, the Canadian public health insurance model offers universal coverage at a much lower cost than the predominately private medical market in the United States.

Many policymakers and pundits celebrate the health-care system as the "jewel in the crown" of the Canadian welfare state. Critics of recent Canadian governments lament the tarnished state of the crown and its lackluster jewel, pointing to serious strains on the system, which are discussed more fully. However, in comparative terms the Canadian health-care system can still be classified among the most successful in the industrialized world. The quality of health-

TABLE 2
Health Expenditure, Selected OECD Countries, 1998

	Total Health Expenditure as % of GDP	Total Health Expenditure per Capita PPP$	Public Expenditure as a % of Total
Australia	8.5	2,043	69.3
Austria	8.2	1,968	70.5
Belgium	8.8	2,081	89.7
Canada	9.5	2,312	69.6
Denmark	8.3	2,133	81.9
Finland	6.9	1,502	76.3
Germany	10.6	2,424	74.6
Italy	8.4	1,783	68.0
Japan	7.6	1,822	78.3
Netherlands	8.6	2,070	70.4
New Zealand	8.1	1,424	77.1
Norway	8.9	2,425	82.8
Sweden	8.4	1,746	83.8
Switzerland	10.4	2,794	73.4
United Kingdom	6.7	1,461	83.7
United States	13.6	4,178	44.7

Source: Organisation for Economic Co-operation and Development, *OECD Health Data 2000: Comparative Analysis of 29 OECD Countries* (Paris: OECD, 2000).

care delivery in Canada ranks among the most sophisticated in the world and the consistent support it enjoys in public opinion polls is remarkable. Until now at least, the Canadian health-care system has also been able to withstand the lure of market incentives and managed care that have led to substantial modifications in the design and delivery of health care in other industrialized countries.[6]

Social scientists tend to classify Canada as a "liberal" welfare state with relatively lower social expenditures than many European countries where the state has a much more extensive role in guaranteeing social protection.[7] But the existence of public, universal health care clearly sets Canada apart from liberal welfare states such as the United States.[8] The Canadian health-care system in effect combines elements of a "liberal" ideology (in that doctors are not employees of the state but rather independent entrepreneurs engaged in a private relationship with their patients) and a more "social democratic" vision (through the public financing of health services and government oversight to ensure equal access to health care). Although this type of system fits the "social insurance" model, the term "national health insurance" is somewhat of a misnomer given the autonomous role of provincial governments in the health sector. A better description is that of provincially regulated health-care systems financed by public revenues, and a federal fiscal contribution tied to the maintenance of certain standards across the provinces.

Historical Development

The initial impetus for the development of public health insurance in Canada came from the combination of provincial innovation with social-democratic politics.[9] It was a provincial government in Saskatchewan, under the leadership of a social-democratic party, that first introduced legislation for public hospital insurance in 1947 and medical insurance in 1962. With these provincial innovations in place, federalism provided the dynamic institutional levers that diffused public hospital and medical insurance across the country as a whole. In 1948, the federal government introduced the National Health Grants Program, which furnished funding for public health and hospital construction in the provinces. However, the federal government soon came under pressure to provide funds to facilitate the implementation of provincial hospital insurance on a Canada-wide basis, and in 1957 it introduced the *Hospital Insurance and Diagnostic Services Act* which allowed for federal sharing of the cost of provincial hospital insurance plans. By 1961, every province in Canada had set up such a plan. In 1962, the Saskatchewan government introduced a further innovation: a medical insurance program that used public funds to reimburse doctors for the services they provided to patients. This again proved to be a successful model and in 1966, the federal government designed another cost-sharing mechanism under the *Medical Care Insurance Act*. By 1971 every province had such a plan in operation and Canada's health insurance system was fully in place.

Although the federal government stipulated that, in order to receive funding, the provinces had to abide by certain conditions in the design of their health-care systems (comprehensive and portable benefits, universal coverage, and public financing), there was substantial scope for provincial programs to reflect regional and local particularities. In the case of Quebec, for example, public health insurance was developed in the context of a larger movement toward social and economic modernization, known as the "Quiet Revolution."[10] Although inspired by social-democratic values and financed in part through federal transfers, Quebec's health-care system, based on integrated health and social services and an emphasis on community care, reflected a specific vision of the role of the state in society.[11]

In 1984, the federal government passed the *Canada Health Act* (CHA). The CHA amalgamated existing federal hospital and medical insurance legislation into a single statute and attempted to assert, in symbolic terms, a substantial role for the federal government in the health-care sector. In more concrete terms, the CHA reinforced the existing conditions regulating health transfers and imposed another, that of "equal access" in order to prohibit practices that could be financial impediments to receiving health-care services. These practices included "extra-billing" (by which physicians charge patients a higher fee than that negotiated with the provincial medical association) and the imposition of user fees in hospitals. Under the CHA, such practices would lead to dollar-for-dollar deductions in the cash portion of federal transfers to the province. The explicit ban on extra-billing and the financial deterrents led to the abolition of the practice in most provinces, although in Ontario, where extra-billing was most widespread, the ban prevailed only after a bitter strike by doctors in 1986.[12] However, as late as 1995, financial penalties were imposed on the government of British Columbia for allowing extra-billing; and as late as 1996, transfers to Alberta were reduced by $1.3 million and to Manitoba by $588,000 because of facility and user fees.

The CHA was, and is, a popular statute and one might conclude that the federal government has the ability to impose necessary deterrents on the provinces. But some provincial governments regard the CHA as violation of the rules of the intergovernmental game and of provincial sovereignty in health care. Quebec, in particular, has long demanded federal withdrawal from areas of provincial jurisdiction, including health care. Intergovernmental relations have been further strained by attempts of the federal government to reduce its fiscal responsibilities in part by reducing the cash transfers to the provinces. All of these developments stand in contrast to the commitment to cooperation (albeit in the closed world of executive level negotiation) that characterized the emergence of health insurance in Canada. Federal cost-sharing plans for hospital and medical insurance were enacted after considerable dialogue with the provinces and formal federal-provincial conferences. Since the 1980s, however, major federal decisions, especially the introduction of the CHA and decisions concerning federal transfers to the provinces, have been made on a unilateral basis, arguably in the context of short-term decisions about public spending rather than on the basis of longer term analyses of the sustainability of the public health-care system.

Financing of Health Care

Public responsibility for the financing of hospitals and reimbursement of medical care is an expensive enterprise for provincial and federal governments alike. As noted earlier, Canada ranks above the Organisation for Economic Co-operation and Development (OECD) average in health expenditures but well below the United States. This spending-to-gross domestic product (GDP) ratio has declined consistently since 1992, when total health spending reached its highest level at 10.2 percent of GDP in Canada. Although hospital operating costs represent the largest share of health-care expenditures, these have declined steadily in the past decade, reflecting the extensive rationalization of provincial hospitals and changes in treatment protocols. In contrast, spending on pharmaceuticals has risen sharply; in fact, drug costs now account for slightly more than physician reimbursement (Table 3). Also noteworthy is that, although provincial health-care systems have so far shut out much of the potential for a widespread private medical market, private spending, whether through supplemental health insurance or direct out-of-pocket payments, has increased steadily over the past two decades. This trend has reflected a number of factors: the increase in drug costs and in the use of outpatient treatments; the de-listing of some previously insured services (such as optometry); and the increase in privately available diagnostic treatment and non-insured technologies such as eye laser surgery and in-vitro fertilization.

TABLE 3
Health Expenditure in Canada

	1977 (%)	1997 (%)
Health Expenditure by Source of Financing		
Provincial spending as % of total health expenditure (includes transfers from the federal government through CHST)	71.6	64.2
Private spending as % of total spending (includes private insurance and out-of-pocket)	23.3	30.6
Federal direct spending	3.1	3.4
Health Expenditure by Use of Funds		
Hospitals	44.1	32.5
Other health-care institutions	10.2	9.9
Physicians	14.7	14.2
Other health professionals	9.6	12.5
Drugs	8.4	14.5
Public health spending	4.6	5.7

Source: Canadian Institute for Health Information, *National Health Expenditure Trends, 1975-1998* (Ottawa: CIHI, 1999).

The public portion of health-care financing comes from government general revenues and not a specific health insurance fund or tax. In other words, governments allocate a certain portion of their yearly budgets to cover the costs of health-care services. Provincial governments and their agencies represent the "single-payer" or "single-tap" through which money flows into the health-care system. This simplifies accounting and administration for health-care providers, but also exposes the health-care industry to the fiscal pressures faced by the public sector in general. Health care accounts for the largest item in provincial budgets and most provinces spend at least 30 percent of their total outlays in this sector (Table 4). For example, in the 1998–99 fiscal year, the Ontario government allocated $19 billion for health care, exactly one-third of its total public expenditure of $57 billion.[13]

The federal government's contribution to provincial health-care funding has declined over the years as the mechanisms for transferring money to the provinces were modified. After 1977, the EPF arrangement distributed money on an equal per capita basis to each province. Increases in the EPF transfer were initially linked to the rate of growth in the economy, but this was reduced to gross national product (GNP) growth minus 2 percent in 1986 and eventually frozen after 1990. In 1995, the EPF arrangement, along with the existing cost-shared Canada Assistance Plan, was replaced by the CHST. The CHST substantially reduced the cash portion of federal transfers to the provinces, although a five-year "cash floor" was subsequently introduced in 1998. These changes have a major impact on the role of the federal government. In the mid-1970s, federal transfers accounted for almost 40 percent of provincial health expenditures; by the mid-1990s, the transfers represented one-third of provincial outlays in health care.[14] In part as a response to public concern about health-care funding, the 1999 federal budget earmarked additional funds to the CHST and introduced measures to eliminate interprovincial disparities. The 1999–2000 budget allocated $28.4 billion to help fund provincial social programs, including health care. The cash portion of the CHST, totaling $14.5 billion, represented 13 percent of total program expenditures by the federal government.[15]

Delivery of Health Care

The health insurance model that has developed in the Canadian provinces is, in comparison to most other countries, a model of surprising simplicity. In contrast to predominantly private health insurance systems, such as in the US, every resident of a province is covered by the same insurance system and no money changes hands at the point of contact between doctor and patient. In comparison to national health systems, such as the UK, doctors and hospitals have remained independent of direct public control by the state. And, unlike social insurance arrangements in Germany in which employers and employees contribute directly to "sickness funds," health care in Canada is financed by general government revenues rather than premiums.

The Canadian model can be summarized by tracing the five principles of the CHA reflected in the design of provincial health-care systems (Figure 1). The first is that of *public administration*. Hospitals are not administered by provincial governments nor are physicians employees of the state; nevertheless, since both hospital and medical services are financed by public money, the providers of health care are considered to be publicly accountable and they remain dependent on political decisions about the allocation of resources. Under the terms of provincial health statutes, these decisions are made by provincial ministries, public medical commissions or, in many provinces, by regional boards acting under the authority of the provincial government. Hospitals are generally operated as non-profit institutions financed by global budgets that are negotiated with provincial governments. They are thus dependent on public funds for most of their operating costs (including medical supplies and equipment) and salaried employees (such as nurses and technicians) and must work within the budgets assigned to them for the fiscal year. The provincial Ministry of Health determines these global budgets although, more recently, allocation decisions in most provinces have become the responsibility of regional boards with representation from government, consumers, and providers. Given the pressure on public expenditures, most hospital operating budgets have been substantially reduced, leading to waiting lists for elective procedures and non-emergency in-patient services and a greater reliance on out-patient care and, in some cases, the closure of hospitals or their transformation into another type of health-care facility. In some provinces, empty hospital wings and privately funded health-care facilities are now used to dispense non-insured benefits. Several well-equipped tertiary care centres are also using excess capacity to treat Americans and other non-Canadians at much higher rates than are charged to provincial residents.

Physicians are reimbursed for their services on a fee-for-service basis through a fee schedule negotiated between provincial governments and provincial medical associations. These fee schedules are roughly similar across the provinces, although there is some variation in the definition of billing codes. The reimbursement is administered by a public agency responsible to the provincial Ministry of Health. These agencies, or commissions, include members of provincial medical associations, government officials, and in some case representatives of consumer groups. In Quebec, the principle of public administration is taken one step further through a system of community health and social service centres known as Centres locaux de services communautaires (CLSC), staffed by salaried physicians. Despite the objection of medical associations, Quebec was also the first province to impose billing limits and caps on specialist salaries, and was one of the first provinces to impose differential fees onto physicians with new billing numbers on the basis of their practice and residence within the province.

The principle of *comprehensiveness*, that all "medically necessary" services should be covered by public health insurance, is defined through the CHA to mean at a minimum all insured services provided by hospitals and doctors. Thus, in all the provinces, most diagnostic, in-patient, and outpatient services are covered, as well as services provided by physicians both in and outside the hospital. Most provinces now specify a range of services that are not covered, such as in-patient incidentals (e.g., private hospital rooms), certain forms of cosmetic surgery, or services supplied by optometrists or chiropractors.

The CHA also states that health benefits should be *universal* in their entitlement and *portable* across provincial boundaries. In other words, every provincial resident is entitled to health-care coverage, regardless of age, income or province of residence. Portability of hospital benefits is guaranteed through reciprocity agreements that allow for direct payment at the provincial rates where the patient is treated. Medically insured benefits are subject to reciprocal agreements between the provinces (except Quebec, which has a lower reimbursement rate and charges non-Quebecers directly for medical services).

The principle of *equal access* means that services should be dispensed on the sole criteria of medical need rather than ability to pay. As noted earlier, the CHA specifies that user fees or extra-billing violate this criterion. Unlike public health insurance systems in other countries, health-care services in the provinces are provided on the basis of first-dollar coverage, without co-payments and without user fees. Also in contrast to many other public systems, Canadians pay for their health-care services through general government taxes on income and consumption rather than contributing to a specific health insurance fund or paying a special tax for health services.

Role of Stakeholders

The preceding description of the delivery of health services reveals an intriguing element of the Canadian model: it is a health-care system in which the "public" financing of costs is combined with "private" delivery of services.[16] Stakeholders, therefore, may hold conflicting values about the health-care system. Patterns of negotiation and compromise among stakeholders likewise reflect a combination of different practices and principles. In comparative terms, the Canadian health-care system has been described as pluralist and entrepreneurial.[17] Like their insured neighbours in the US, consumers of care in Canada have relative freedom to choose their health-care providers. Canadian physicians function as private entrepreneurs in much the same way as many American physicians do; indeed, given the proliferation of managed care arrangements in the US perhaps even more so. Influential groups, primarily physicians, but also organized labour, business, and consumer groups, play an important role in the policy-making arena. Some corporatist patterns are also evident: for example, as in Germany or France, institutionalized fee schedule negotiations between peak physician associations and provincial governments determine reimbursement rates for medical services. And, while hospitals remain independent, non-profit institutions, government agencies or regional boards are responsible for allocating global budgets.

The primary stakeholders in any health-care system are the consumers of care. Among Canadians, it is clear that there still exists enduring support for public health care and the CHA principles. As federal and provincial politicians have learned to their peril, electoral campaigns are more effective when designed around promises to sustain public health insurance rather than dismantle it. Every major political party, regardless of how opaquely worded the message may be, supports in some way the idea that health care is a public good. Although health care was not a principal issue in the 2000 election, the campaign did reveal that "two-tier" health care — the coexistence of private and public insurance systems for core health services — still has a negative connotation in Canada. In many provinces, public protest over expenditure cuts that adversely affected the delivery of health-care services prompted lawmakers to rethink their cost-cutting strategies.

In general, public opinion toward health care is based primarily on the satisfaction, or dissatisfaction, of one's experience with the delivery of health care. Polls commissioned by the National Forum on Health found that Canadians are profoundly attached to equality and universality in health care.[18] Comparative polls that ask respondents to rate their health-care systems against those of other countries also demonstrated a widespread confidence among Canadians in the 1980s and early 1990s.[19] More recently, however, some thought-provoking trends have developed in Canadians' attitudes toward their health-care system. There is, for example, a growing dissatisfaction with quality of services and access to care. Opinion polls show negative reactions to many provincial health-reform initiatives such as expenditure cuts and the rationalization of the hospital sector. For example, a 1998 Angus Reid poll found that 46 percent of Canadians thought recent health reforms compromised the quality of service. More profound in this respect is the revelation of a growing unease about the future sustainability of the health-care system. In 1988, cross-national studies showed that only 5 percent of Canadians agreed that their health-care system had to be "rebuilt completely"; by 1998, this figure had increased to 23 percent.[20] (See Table 6). But public opinion shows paradoxical trends about what this means exactly. Some polls find support for user fees, for example, but at the same time reveal support for federal standards.[21]

The diffuse interests of consumers can be contrasted with the more specific interests of provider groups. Stakeholders such as hospital workers, doctors, insurers, and hospital administrators have different — and potentially conflicting — interests in the health-care system. As public sector employees, salaried hospital personnel have been the most affected by cost-control measures. Provincial nurses' associations have become especially vocal, even resorting to strike action, in protesting cuts to public funding because of the threat to job security and the deterioration of workplace quality. With the closure of hospitals and cuts to public funding in the past decade, many nurses have chosen to vote with their feet and relocate to higher paying positions in the United States.

The migration of Canadian nurses and physicians to the US has fuelled concerns about the so-called "brain drain" of health-care providers. In 1996, for example, 30 percent of medical school graduates in Canada chose to practise outside the country.[22] Like nurses, physicians have divided interests. On the one hand, the public health-care system has allowed Canadian doctors to retain fee-for-service medicine, a practice increasingly threatened in the United States because of the proliferation of managed care arrangements. As a founding member of the Health Action Lobby, for example, the Canadian Medical Association (CMA) has insisted on more stable federal funding of provincial health-care systems. On the other hand, while some physicians may hold deep convictions about public health insurance, support for such a system is generally based on the potential to reap a measure of economic benefit from it. For most doctors, particularly specialists, reductions in health expenditures and restrictions on fees and billing jeopardize this. The CMA and many of its provincial affiliates, most notably in Alberta, British Columbia, and Ontario, have argued that, in light of continued cuts to public funding, the principles of the *Canada Health Act* are unsustainable. In the past few years, CMA general meetings have been open forums of debate over the desirability of private medicine and market incentives in Canada. While resolutions on this issue have been narrowly defeated at these meetings, they have gained considerable currency within the medical community. The CMA has advocated a public debate on private alternatives to health care and CMA polls suggest that 70 percent of Canadian doctors favour a two-tier health-care system.[23]

Since the advent of public health insurance, private insurers have been relatively minor players at the margin of the health-care system in Canada. The vast majority of private health insurance consists of supplementary coverage (limited to services not covered by the public system) provided through employer-based group policies. With more and more discussion of parallel private financing of health care, the future of the private insurance industry presents a conundrum. For the supporters of public health insurance, expanding the role of private insurers will lead to the same problems as those facing the US, namely administrative waste, risk-selection of individuals and potentially the undermining of support for the public system.[24] Many insurers — and the employers they contract with — are cautious about expanding private health insurance options given the strength of the existing public system.[25] Still, as private expenditures continue to increase and as provincial governments continue to restructure the health-care system, private insurers, particularly the new breed of multinationals that have entered the Canadian market in the 1990s, seem poised to play a larger, more aggressive role in health-reform debates. Unlike many other social services, the existence of private insurance provides the potential for concrete alternatives to the public sector.

Finally, governments can also be considered stakeholders in the health-care system. Provincial governments have a central and obvious role to play in regulating and financing health care. This role is a difficult one, however, because it involves both a commitment to the existing system and a recognition of heavy financial considerations. The federal government, meanwhile, plays a technically more limited role (through fiscal transfers) but a disproportionately more important symbolic role via the CHA. Despite provincial complaints of interference and insufficient funding, the federal government has been able to retain a politically rewarding niche as the "guardian" of a popular public health-care system.

FEDERALISM AND HEALTH CARE

In comparative context, Canada is among the more decentralized of federations.[26] Australia and the United States, for example, offer examples of more centralized models in which the federal government exerts a much more visible, and tangible, role in health matters than do the states. Federal legislation in Germany must pass muster in the Bundesrat, but the individual Länder have little formal authority in health policy. In Canada, the federal government has a limited formal role in the health-care sector. Health policy remains the exclusive jurisdiction of the provinces and provincial governments make the principal decisions that affect the design of health-care services and the allocation of health-care resources. From the point of view of real politics, however, both levels of government are responsible for the functioning of the health-care system and, ultimately, bear the burden for its successes and failures. The ascendance of health-care issues to the front and centre of the political agenda, both national and provincial, has increased the potential for political conflict about roles and resources.

Federalism is usually considered an institutional constraint in social policy-making because of the difficulty of achieving consensus in a system of divided powers.[27] Jurisdictional conflict did contribute to delays in health-care reform as part of a broader postwar social security program in Canada, and resistance from Ontario and Quebec to the use of the federal spending power initially stymied federal initiatives in this area. By the same token, however, Canadian federalism provided the potential for experimentation and expansion in health-care protection.[28] The passage of landmark hospital and medical insurance legislation designed in Saskatchewan illustrates how the federal system encouraged laboratories of innovations. But the "semi-centralized" features of Canadian federalism, in particular the important fiscal role of the federal government, also reveal how federalism can encourage the effective diffusion of such innovation across the country.[29]

Although interregional disparities are also apparent in unitary systems, federalism does raise the problem of how to guarantee a measure of uniformity across disparate political and economic units.[30] In Canada, the use of the federal spending power has tended to mitigate, although not resolve, this problem in the health-care sector and the federal government continues to exercise some pressure on provincial policy design through the norms enunciated in the CHA. Despite this counterweight to decentralization, however, Canadian federalism has been flexible enough to accommodate considerable regional variation, as exemplified by the unique design of Quebec's health-care system. Moreover, although Quebec does not always attend "executive" level intergovernmental meetings of provincial health ministers and their federal counterpart, all provinces participate in the dozens of existing intergovernmental health advisory committees that cover everything from population wellness to physician supply.

Divided responsibilities can also create potential hazards and road-blocks to efficient health policy outcomes. Intergovernmental disputes or disagreements can present a brake to rapid change, delaying the passage of legislation or leading to factional struggles over reform options. Such disputes are not necessarily disadvantageous in a liberal democracy, since they bring political struggles about resource allocation into the public domain. Nevertheless, the multiplicity of stakeholder interests in a federal setting and the use of health care as a political football between governments complicates efforts to coherently address problems in health-care provision and financing. The lack of coordinated consultative mechanisms for health-care funding, for example, reveal an accountability problem that makes it difficult to assume responsibility and to assign blame within the health policy community. The failure of existing intergovernmental arrangements to allay concerns about the viability of the Canadian health-care model has allowed ample room for the emergence of new alternatives in public debate about health reform.

Intergovernmental disputes in health care have centred on the perceived interference of the federal government in a provincial domain and the allocation of federal transfers to the provinces. Although shared-cost programs in hospital and medical insurance initially involved federal accounting oversight to determine the amounts of money to send to the provinces, the shift to block-funding through EPF in 1977 allowed the provinces more flexibility in their financial arrangements. However, there was a long-term downside to block-funding for the provinces. Because growth in the federal transfer under EPF was tied to growth in the economy rather than actual provincial health expenditures, the provincial governments bore the brunt of rapid increases in health-care costs during subsequent decades. Moreover, with the passage of the CHA in 1984, the federal government made it clear that provincial flexibility was still constrained by the existence of a set of health policy principles and a dispute resolution mechanism that allows for little provincial participation. If the federal minister of health finds that a province does not respect a CHA principle, he or she can inform the Cabinet and ask that deductions be made from federal payments. Although there is consultation between the federal minister and the province, there is relatively little room for negotiation or dispute resolution. This process gives the federal minister of health the potential to act as "judge and jury" in disputes with the provinces in a policy sector that is under provincial jurisdiction.[31] With the introduction of the CHST in 1995 and substantial reductions in federal transfers to the provinces, intergovernmental disputes over health care intensified.

Taken together, these points of contention have led to uneasiness about the boundaries between federal and provincial responsibilities in health care.

The sense that the rules of the game were changed unilaterally has been reinforced by the ideological disposition of Conservative governments in Ontario and Alberta, concern among centre-left governments at the way in which health policy decisions were being effected by the federal Department of Finance, and the perennial quest for autonomy by Quebec. These dynamics have spurred provincial leaders to engage in discussions about forging a new partnership for social reform. At the 1995 Annual Premiers' Conference, the premiers declared their intention to take a leadership role in social policy reform, including a process of joint federal-provincial control over the CHA. Premiers demanded federal-provincial consultations to interpret the CHA and resolve disputes over its meaning, and a predictable funding base for health services. In 1997, the provinces reaffirmed their insistence that an effective partnership between federal and provincial governments would entail "adequate, predictable and stable cash transfers" and formal mechanisms to ensure more transparency in dispute resolution.[32] In August 1998, all ten provincial premiers (including Quebec) reached agreement on how to adapt intergovernmental processes to reflect provincial interests and needs. These included the possibility of opting out of federal social spending programs; the joint administration of any federal-provincial programs (including dispute resolution); and a stipulation that the federal government must obtain majority provincial consent before initiating new spending programs.

In an attempt to regain leadership in the intergovernmental arena, the federal government invited the premiers to join a "social union" that could build a new flexibility into the Canadian federation. The final agreement between the two orders of government fell far short of the provinces' demands. The new framework agreement, signed by all the provinces except Quebec in February 1999, did acknowledge the need for provincial input in shared-cost programs and dispute resolution, but did not provide for opting-out. The federal government also responded in financial terms. The 1999 federal budget, unveiled one week later, announced the injection of $11.5 billion over five years to health transfers to the provinces in an attempt to demonstrate the federal government's renewed commitment to providing predictable funding for public health care in the provinces. In anticipation of the general election campaign in the fall of 2000, the federal government committed an additional $21.1 billion to CHST payments to the provinces over five years, plus $2.3 billion for funding priorities in primary care, health information technology, and medical equipment.

Despite this new injection of money by the federal government, intergovernmental sparring continues unabated. Much of this conflict is inevitable given the variety of ideologies and interests at play in Canada's political system. While public shouting matches between governments are not a novelty in Canadian politics, tensions have deepened, revealing a more diffuse but potentially more explosive malaise about federalism and health policy. Squabbles over money are now overshadowed by more substantial conflict about the extent to which the federal government can impose rules about health policy in the absence of fiscal muscle to enforce them.

IMPACT OF FEDERALISM ON THE PROVISION OF HEALTH CARE

Despite the fact that health care in Canada falls under the auspices of ten provincial and two territorial health insurance plans, there is considerable symmetry in terms of the level of benefits and amounts of money spent on health between regions in the country. The provisions of the CHA and the transfer of federal funds, in addition to interprovincial agreements on reciprocal hospital and medical services ensure this relative symmetry.

In general, Canadians receive the same health-care benefits regardless of where they reside in Canada. A cursory reading of provincial health statutes or the annual reports submitted to the federal government shows that, in each case, virtually 100 percent of the eligible population is covered for all medically necessary procedures on equal terms and conditions. The differences in coverage that exist tend to be minimal. For example, optometry and some chiropractic services are covered in British Columbia and Ontario, but not in Quebec. In addition, prescription drug coverage can vary, as some provinces subsidize the costs for the elderly and poor or offer a supplementary pharmacare program. However, Tables 4 and 6 demonstrate that the federal transfers and equalization payments tend to offset the impact of differences in the economic wealth of regions on the health services enjoyed by their residents. Table 4 shows that per capita health-care spending is fairly similar across the provinces (although substantially higher in the northern territories where all activities are more expensive); and Table 6 confirms that the poorer provinces of Atlantic Canada (Newfoundland, Prince Edward Island, Nova Scotia, and New Brunswick) are not disadvantaged in terms of the number of doctors, nurses, and acute-care hospital beds per 1,000 population.

Some disparities remain, of course, both within and between provinces. Provinces with lower average incomes tend to have more difficulty in attracting

TABLE 4
Health Expenditures in the Provinces and Territories, 1998

	Government Health Expenditures as % of Provincial GDP	*Provincial Health Expenditures as % of Total Gov't Program*	*Total Health Spending per capita ($)*
Newfoundland	9.1	31.9	2,685
Prince Edward Island	7.5	29.3	2,599
Nova Scotia	8.0	39.2	2,732
New Brunswick	7.1	30.4	2,548
Quebec	6.4	30.3	2,586
Ontario	5.3	37.6	2,875
Manitoba	6.8	34.8	2,875
Saskatchewan	6.1	37.0	2,738
Alberta	4.4	33.2	2,707
British Columbia	6.8	33.5	2,898
Yukon	6.5	15.1	3,326
Northwest Territories	9.4	17.3	5,244
Canada Average	5.8	34.0	2,776

Source: Canadian Institute for Health Information, *National Health Expenditure Trends, 1975-1998* (Ottawa: CIHI, 1999).

FIGURE 1
Canada Health Act, 1984

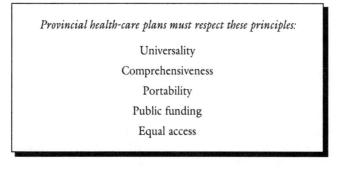

Provincial health-care plans must respect these principles:

Universality

Comprehensiveness

Portability

Public funding

Equal access

TABLE 5
Canadian Public Opinion in Comparative Perspective

	System Needs to be Rebuilt		System Needs Minor Changes	
	1988 (%)	1998 (%)	1988 (%)	1998 (%)
Canada	5	23	56	20
United States	29	33	10	17
United Kingdom	17	14	27	25
Australia	17	30	34	18

Source: Karen Donelan *et al.*, "The Cost of Health System Change: Public Discontent in Five Nations," *Health Affairs* 18, 3(1999):206-16; Commonwealth Fund, *1998 Commonwealth Fund International Health Policy Survey*, Survey conducted by Louis Harris and Associates Inc., Study No. 728346 (New York: The Commonwealth Fund, 1998).

TABLE 6
Health Services in the Provinces and Territories, 1998

	Doctors per 1,000 Population	Registered Nurses per 1,000 Population	Acute-Care Hospital Beds per 1,000 Population
Newfoundland	1.7	9.8	3.3
Prince Edward Island	1.3	9.3	3.5
Nova Scotia	1.9	9.1	3.6
New Brunswick	1.5	9.9	3.9
Quebec	2.1	7.7	3.7
Ontario	1.8	6.9	2.2
Manitoba	1.7	8.9	3.6
Saskatchewan	1.5	8.2	3.9
Alberta	1.6	7.5	2.2
British Columbia	1.9	6.9	2.2
Yukon	1.5	7.8	1.8
Northwest Territories	0.9	7.8	3.9

Source: Canadian Institute for Health Information, *National Health Expenditure Trends, 1975-1998* (Ottawa: CIHI, 1999); Health Canada, *Canada Health Act Annual Report, 1997-98* (Ottawa: Supply and Services Canada, 1998).

and keeping highly-qualified physicians; this is of particular importance in the Atlantic provinces, where the concentration of specialists tends to be lower than in larger provinces such as Ontario and Quebec. Less populated regions and more remote areas have similar concerns. In the northern territories, for example, the small number of available specialists and acute-care hospitals mean that patients must often travel to urban health-care facilities in the south. In most provinces, the major disparities in physician ratios and available facilities are between urban centres and "underserviced areas" in rural communities. This has led to several rural incentive programs designed to attract physicians to these areas, with mixed success.[33] In addition, most provinces attempt to impose financial penalties on new physicians who set up practice in overserviced areas in major urban centres. The latter initiatives may become a contentious issue, however, and the courts have increasingly stepped into the health policy field. The BC Supreme Court upheld the challenge launched by three doctors trained in Ontario protesting the differential fees for new billing numbers on the basis of mobility rights under section 6 of the Canadian Charter of Rights and Freedoms. In this case, the provisions of the Charter call into question the ability of provincial governments to implement policy initiatives.[34]

Attempts at cost control in the provinces raise larger issues about the sustainability of public financing of the health-care sector and the extent to which the federal government can expect provinces to respect the CHA in future health reform. As we have seen, provincial governments have complained bitterly about the reduction in federal transfers, beginning with EPF in the 1980s and the CHST arrangements after 1995. Charges of "off-loading" the federal deficit onto the provinces underlined the fiscal crunch many provinces found themselves in, attempting to fund expensive health-care services with reduced federal money. Concerns were also raised about whether existing standards could be "enforced" under the CHA without adequate financial incentive. Although the 1999 budget and the injection of new federal money in 2000 mollified some critics, two essential questions remain. The first is whether federal involvement inhibits provincial attempts at health-care reform. For example, the Alberta government has expressed interest in encouraging market forces in the health-care system, and tabled legislation in 1999 to allow private clinics and surgical facilities to deal with excess demand for services,[35] a move challenged by the federal government which considers such private clinics a threat to equality of access to health-care services. The second question lies at the heart of the federal-provincial debate: is the CHA necessary to ensure a common level of benefits across the provinces and territories, or is interprovincial cooperation a better way to frame the parameters of the health-care system? It is difficult to envision what the health-care system would look like without federal involvement. It is probably safe to say that public opinion would play a large role in convincing governments to maintain broadly universal health-care systems. However, it is more difficult to be certain that these systems would function in the same way in terms of their financing and administration. In a policy sector such as health, where the incentive to retain jurisdictional sovereignty is high and the economic costs of non-cooperation are low, some provinces might be tempted to design increasingly disparate health-reform scenarios.

There is no denying that the health-care system occupies an influential symbolic role in Canadian federalism. The success of public health insurance provides a yardstick by which many Canadians compare themselves to the rest of the world, in particular the United States. In no other country are citizens so readily inclined to equate their values with a social program as Canadians do when asserting that health care is "an essential part of their national identity."[36] Canadians remain committed to the five principles of the CHA and, in so doing, to the federal presence in the health-care sector. The federal government, in turn, has many reasons for wanting to maintain this presence, including the ability to ensure common benefits for all Canadians, and the lucrative political rewards of occupying a visible space in this popular policy sector.

CONCLUSION

Federalism is a defining feature of the Canadian health-care model. The provisions of the *Constitution Act* and the efforts of activist provincial governments provided the impetus for public health insurance. Provincial innovation combined with cooperative intergovernmental relations in the 1950s and 1960s facilitated the expansion of health benefits and the development of the Canadian welfare state. The existing mosaic of ten provincial and three territorial health-care systems reflects the best of what federalism can achieve in Canada: meaningful decentralization and relative financial autonomy combined with a measure of functional symmetry and regional equity.

The dynamics of Canadian federalism have contributed to the development of a remarkably successful health-care model. The flexibility of Canadian federalism, in particular jurisdictional decentralization toward the provinces, has allowed substantial variation in health-care delivery systems and policy initiatives tailored to the particular economic and social situations of disparate provinces and regions. Provincial and territorial governments administer their own health insurance programs and have autonomous power to allocate money and resources through the system. Attempts to reorganize hospital resources, manage physician supply, and regionalize certain decision-making processes are all examples of how the provinces exert considerable autonomy in health reform, without the central government oversight that is the norm in other federal systems.

The presence of the federal government does impose certain constraints on provincial governments. So far, the federal government has used its fiscal and symbolic role as a means to ensure the integrity of the Canadian health-care model, without having to shoulder the lion's share of financial and administrative burdens. The use of the spending power combined with the "enforcement" of the CHA gives the federal government the ability to set the boundaries of health reform, ensure compatibility among provincial health-care systems, and act as a deterrent to market-based experimentation. Thus, despite *de jure* decentralization, the federal government binds together provincial health-care systems in a way that goes beyond the situation in many unitary states where recent reforms have led to considerable interregional differences in the financing and delivery of health services.

As intergovernmental relations evolve and change the institutional boundaries in health policy-making, the binding function of the federal government may be unravelling. In the past decade the federal government has decreased its fiscal responsibilities toward the provincial health-care systems while simultaneously attempting to expand its political space through the CHA. Provincial governments, meanwhile, have grown more impatient with the federal government on issues of fiscal transfers and (particularly in the case of Quebec) questions of jurisdictional boundaries in health and social policy. These centrifugal pressures have intensified as private market alternatives become more visible in the health-care sector. In this context, it seems unlikely that the provincial innovations of the first decades of the twenty-first century will resemble those of Saskatchewan or Quebec in the twentieth century.

NOTES

[1]Paul E. Peterson, *City Limits* (Chicago: University of Chicago Press, 1981).
[2]See Kenneth C. Wheare, *Federal Government*, 2d ed. (London: Oxford University Press, 1951).
[3]Dennis Guest, *The Emergence of Social Security in Canada*, 3d ed. (Vancouver: University of British Columbia Press, 1997).
[4]Donald Smiley, ed., *The Rowell-Sirois Report*, Book 1 (Toronto: McClelland & Stewart).
[5]See Antonia Maioni, *Parting at the Crossroads: The Emergence of Health Insurance in the United States and Canada* (Princeton, NJ: Princeton University Press, 1998).
[6]Antonia Maioni, "Market Incentives and Health Reform in Canada," Working Paper No. 99/12 (Florence: European University Institute, 1999).
[7]G. Esping-Andersen, *The Three Worlds of Welfare Capitalism* (Princeton, NJ: Princeton University Press, 1990).
[8]See Robert T. Kudrle and Theodore R. Marmor, "The Development of Welfare States in North America," in *The Development of Welfare States in Europe and America*, ed. P. Flora and A. Heidenheimer (New Brunswick, NJ: Transaction Books).
[9]Maioni, *Parting at the Crossroads*.
[10]See Kenneth McRoberts, *Quebec: Social Change and Political Crisis*, 3d ed. (Toronto: Oxford University Press, 1993).
[11]Pierre Bergeron and France Gagnon, "La prise en charge étatique de la santé au Québec," in *Le Système de santé au Québec: Organisations, acteurs et enjeux*, ed. V. Lemieux *et al.* (Sainte-Foy: Lew Presses de l'Université Laval, 1994).
[12]Carolyn Tuohy, "Medicine and the State in Canada: The Extra-Billing Issue in Perspective," *Canadian Journal of Political Science* 23, 2 (1988):267-96.
[13]Ontario, Ministry of Finance, *Public Accounts in Ontario 1999-2000*, Vol. 1 (Toronto: Government of Ontario).
[14]Canadian Institute for Health Information, *National Health Expenditure Trends, 1975-1998* (Ottawa: CIHI, 1999).
[15]Canada. Department of Finance, *Federal Transfers to Provinces and Territories* (Ottawa: Supply and Services Canada, 1999).
[16]C. David Naylor, *Private Practice, Public Payment: Canadian Medicine and the Politics of Health Insurance, 1911-1966* (Montreal and Kingston: McGill-Queen's University Press, 1986).
[17]Charles F. Andrain, *Public Health Policies and Social Inequality* (New York: New York University Press, 1998).
[18]National Forum on Health, *Canada Health Action: Building on the Legacy* (Ottawa: Minister of Public Works and Government Services, 1997).
[19]Robert Blendon *et al.*, "Satisfaction with Health Systems in Ten Nations," *Health Affairs* 9, 2 (1990):185-92.

[20]Karen Donelan *et al.*, "The Cost of Health System Change: Public Discontent in Five Nations," *Health Affairs* 18, 3 (1999):206-16.

[21]Suzanne Peters, *Explaining Canadian Values: Foundations for Well-Being*, Study No. F-01 (Ottawa: Canadian Policy Research Network, 1995).

[22]Charlotte Gray, "How Bad is the Brain Drain?" *Canadian Medical Association Journal* 161, 8 (1999):1028-29.

[23]Charlotte Gray, "Visions of our Health Care Future: Is a Parallel Private System the Answer?" *Canadian Medical Association Journal* 154 (1996):1084-87.

[24]Robert G. Evans, "Going for the Gold: The Redistributive Agenda Behind Market-Based Health Care Reform," *Journal of Health Politics, Policy and Law* 22, 2 (1997):475-96.

[25]Raisa Deber *et al.*, "Why Not Private Health Insurance?: Actuarial Principles Meet Provider Dreams," *Canadian Medical Association Journal* 161, 5 (1999):545-47.

[26]Ronald L. Watts, *Comparing Federal Systems*, 2d ed. (Kingston and Montreal: School of Policy Studies, Queen's University and McGill-Queen's University Press, 1999).

[27]Keith G. Banting, *The Welfare State and Canadian Federalism*, 2d ed. (Kingston and Montreal: McGill-Queen's University Press, 1987).

[28]Carolyn Tuohy, "Federalism and Canadian Health Care Policy," in *Challenges to Federalism: Policy-Making in Canada and the Federal Republic of Germany*, ed. W. Chandler and C. Zollner (Kingston: Institute of Intergovernmental Relations, Queen's University, 1989); Gwendolyn Gray, *Federalism and Health Policy: The Development of Health Systems in Canada and Australia* (Toronto: University of Toronto Press, 1991).

[29]Keith G. Banting, "The Past Speaks to the Future: Lessons from the Postwar Social Union," in *Canada — The State of the Federation 1997: Non-Constitutional Renewal*, ed. H. Lazar (Kingston: Institute of Intergovernmental Relations, Queen's University, 1998).

[30]Franca Maino and Antonia Maioni, *Fiscal Federalism and Health Care Reform in Canada and Italy*, Quaderni di scienza dell'amministrazione e politiche pubbliche, Università di Pavia, 4/99.

[31]Ministerial Council on Social Policy Reform and Renewal, *Report to Premiers* (Ottawa: Supply and Services Canada, 1995), p. 17.

[32]Conference of Provincial/Territorial Ministers of Health, *Renewed Vision for Canada's Health System* (Halifax: The Council, 1997).

[33]Peter Hutten-Czapski, "Rural Incentive Programs: A Failing Report Card," *Canadian Medical Association Journal* 3, 4 (1998):242-47.

[34]Christopher P. Manfredi and Antonia Maioni, "Judicial Management of Provincial Health Care Policy." Paper given at meeting of Canadian Political Science Association, Ottawa, 31 May 1998.

[35]Alberta, Department of Health and Wellness, *Policy Statement on the Delivery of Surgical Services*, 17 November 1999.

[36]National Forum on Health, *Canada Health Action.*

Queen's Policy Studies
Recent Publications

The Queen's Policy Studies Series is dedicated to the exploration of major policy issues that confront governments in Canada and other western nations. McGill-Queen's University Press is the exclusive world representative and distributor of books in the series.

School of Policy Studies

Governing Food: Science, Safety and Trade, Peter W. B. Phillips and Robert Wolfe (eds.), 2001
Paper ISBN 0-88911-897-3 Cloth ISBN 0-88911-903-1

The Nonprofit Sector and Government in a New Century, Kathy L. Brock and Keith G. Banting (eds.), 2001
Paper ISBN 0-88911-901-5 Cloth ISBN 0-88911-905-8

The Dynamics of Decentralization: Canadian Federalism and British Devolution, Trevor C. Salmon and Michael Keating (eds.), 2001 ISBN 0-88911-895-7

Innovation, Institutions and Territory: Regional Innovation Systems in Canada, J. Adam Holbrook and David A. Wolfe (eds.), 2000 Paper ISBN 0-88911-891-4 Cloth ISBN 0-88911-893-0

Backbone of the Army: Non-Commissioned Officers in the Future Army, Douglas L. Bland (ed.), 2000
ISBN 0-88911-889-2

Precarious Values: Organizations, Politics and Labour Market Policy in Ontario, Thomas R. Klassen, 2000
Paper ISBN 0-88911-883-3 Cloth ISBN 0-88911-885-X

The Nonprofit Sector in Canada: Roles and Relationships, Keith G. Banting (ed.), 2000
Paper ISBN 0-88911-813-2 Cloth ISBN 0-88911-815-9

Institute of Intergovernmental Relations

Disability and Federalism: Comparing Different Approaches to Full Participation, David Cameron and Fraser Valentine (ed.), 2001 Paper ISBN 0-88911-857-4 Cloth ISBN 0-88911-867-1, ISBN 0-88911-845-0 (set)

Federalism, Democracy and Health Policy in Canada, Duane Adams (ed.), 2001
Paper ISBN 0-88911-853-1 Cloth ISBN 0-88911-865-5, ISBN 0-88911-845-0 (set)

Federalism, Democracy and Labour Market Policy in Canada, Tom McIntosh (ed.), 2000
ISBN 0-88911-849-3, ISBN 0-88911-845-0 (set)

Canada: The State of the Federation 1999/2000, vol. 14, *Toward a New Mission Statement for Canadian Fiscal Federalism,* Harvey Lazar (ed.), 2000 Paper ISBN 0-88911-843-4 Cloth ISBN 0-88911-839-6

Canada: The State of the Federation 1998/99, vol. 13, *How Canadians Connect,* Harvey Lazar and Tom McIntosh (eds.), 1999 Paper ISBN 0-88911-781-0 Cloth ISBN 0-88911-779-9

Managing the Environmental Union: Intergovernmental Relations and Environmental Policy in Canada, Patrick C. Fafard and Kathryn Harrison (eds.), 2000 ISBN 0-88911-837-X

Stretching the Federation: The Art of the State in Canada, Robert Young (ed.), 1999 ISBN 0-88911-777-2

Comparing Federal Systems, 2d ed., Ronald L. Watts, 1999 ISBN 0-88911-835-3

John Deutsch Institute for the Study of Economic Policy

The State of Economics in Canada: Festschrift in Honour of David Slater, Patrick Grady and Andrew Sharpe (eds.), 2001 Paper ISBN 0-88911-942-2 Cloth ISBN 0-88911-940-6

The 2000 Federal Budget, Paul A.R. Hobson (ed.), Policy Forum Series no. 37, 2001
Paper ISBN 0-88911-816-7 Cloth ISBN 0-88911-814-0

Room to Manoeuvre? Globalization and Policy Convergence, Thomas J. Courchene (ed.),
Bell Canada Papers no. 6, 1999 Paper ISBN 0-88911-812-4 Cloth ISBN 0-88911-812-4

Women and Work, Richard P. Chaykowski and Lisa M. Powell (eds.), 1999
Paper ISBN 0-88911-808-6 Cloth ISBN 0-88911-806-X

Available from: McGill-Queen's University Press
Tel: 1-800-387-0141 (ON and QC excluding Northwestern ON)
1-800-387-0172 (all other provinces and Northwestern ON)
E-mail: customer.service@ccmailgw.genpub.com

Institute of Intergovernmental Relations
Recent Publications

The Spending Power in Federal Systems: A Comparative Study by Ronald L. Watts, 1999
ISBN 0-88911-829-9

Étude comparative du pouvoir de dépenser dans d'autres régimes fédéraux par Ronald L. Watts, 1999
ISBN 0-88911-831-0

*Constitutional Patriation: The Lougheed-Lévesque Correspondence/Le rapatriement de la
Constitution: La correspondance de Lougheed et Lévesque*, with an Introduction by
J. Peter Meekison/avec une introduction de J. Peter Meekison, 1999   ISBN 0-88911-833-7

Securing the Social Union: A Commentary on the Decentralized Approach, Steven A. Kennett, 1998
ISBN 0-88911-767-5

Working Paper Series

2001

1. *Tax Competition and the Fiscal Union: Balancing Competition and Harmonization in Canada.*
Proceedings of a Symposium held 9-10 June 2000, edited by Douglas Brown, Queen's University

2. *Federal Occupational Training Policy: A Neo-Institutionalist Analysis* by Gordon DiGiacomo,
Consultant in Workplace Relations, Greely, Ontario

3. *Federalism and Labour Market Policy in Germany and Canada: Exploring the Path Dependency of
Reforms in the 1990s* by Thomas R. Klassen, Trent University and Steffen Schneider, University of
Augsburg, Germany

4. *Bifurcated and Integrated Parties in Parliamentary Federations: The Canadian and German Cases*
by Wolfgang Renzsch, Otto-von-Guericke Universität Magdeburg, Germany

5. *The Two British Columbias* by Phillip Resnick, University of British Columbia and *The West Wants
In! (But What is the West? and What is "In?")* by Peter McCormick, University of Lethbridge

6. *Federalism and Labour Policy in Canada* by Gordon DiGiacomo

7. *Quebec's Place in the Canada of the Future* by Benoît Pelletier

8. *The Evolution of Support for Sovereignty – Myths and Realities*, by Claire Durand, Université de
Montréal

2000

1. *The Agreement on Internal Trade: An Institutional Response to Changing Conceptions, Roles and
Functions in Canadian Federalism* by Howard Leeson, University of Regina

1999

1. *Processes of Constitutional Restructuring: The Canadian Experience in Comparative Context*
by Ronald L. Watts, Queen's University

2. *Parliament, Intergovernmental Relations and National Unity* by C.E.S. Franks, Queen's University

3. *The United Kingdom as a Quasi-Federal State* by Gerard Hogan, Queen's University

4. *The Federal Spending Power in Canada: Nation-Building or Nation-Destroying?* by Hamish
Telford, Queen's University

For a complete list of working papers see: www.iigr.ca

These publications are available from:
Institute of Intergovernmental Relations, Queen's University, Kingston, Ontario K7L 3N6
Tel: (613) 533-2080 / Fax: (613) 533-6868; E-mail: iigr@qsilver.queensu.ca